How to be

EQUINE
VETERINARIAN

A Guide for Teens

JUSTIN B. LONG

ERICA LACHER, DVM

Published in the United States by Springhill Media
Gainesville, FL

SPRINGHILL

eBook ISBN: 978-1-948169-37-0
Paperback ISBN: 978-1-948169-38-7

Library of Congress Control Number: 2020903715

CONTENTS

INTRODUCTION

So, you want to be a horse vet. Or, it seems like a pretty good idea, but you're not 100% positive about it. That's okay! This is the time to figure these things out, and this book will give you some of the tools you'll need along the way.

The path to becoming a veterinarian is long and difficult. We're not telling you this to scare you away, but we want you to know that it requires a lot of hard work. Once you become a veterinarian, the hard work continues. Horse vets work long hours, and it's usually outside. That means if it's raining, you're getting wet. If it's hot, you're hot. If it's cold, you'd better be dressed for it. Being an equine veterinarian isn't a job. It's a lifestyle. If you're already a horse person, then you're familiar with it, at least to a degree.

This book is broken down into sections to make it easier to digest. If you think you want to be an equine veterinarian, then there is a process you need to go through. We've arranged this book starting at the beginning of this process, when you're just starting high school. If you're already in or past high school and trying to catch up, that's okay!

You'll just have to work smarter with the time you've got. We can't guarantee that you'll get into vet school by following these guidelines. No one can guarantee that. However, you will definitely be a much stronger candidate if you do.

Speaking of time: this is a topic we will keep coming back to. Time is your most valuable resource. Between now and the day you get into vet school, what you do with your time is a big deal. Don't worry, we'll cover all of that. Just know that time management can't be over-emphasized. Poor time management skills in college keep some people from getting into vet school, so we're going to help you avoid that pitfall.

The information in this book comes from a variety of sources. Aside from Dr. Lacher, who is a practicing equine veterinarian and business owner, and is on the admissions committee for the University of Florida vet school, we've talked to a lot of people who are at various stages in their journey. Some are practicing veterinarians.

Some are interns, fresh out of vet school. Some are vet students. Some are veterinary technicians who are in college, or recently graduated, and are still trying to get into vet school. Some are undergrad students who haven't even applied to vet school yet. This gives you relevant feedback from people who are on the same journey you want to take, and from every aspect of it.

We decided to write this guide for a lot of reasons. For one thing, we need more equine veterinarians. There are more horses than ever, and fewer and fewer veterinarians taking care of them. It's also very challenging to get into vet school, and you need every resource you can get. Many eager students arrive at college, having done none of the things they needed to do prior to getting there to set them up for a successful vet school application process. With this book, you'll be able to map out your path and arrive prepared and experienced.

The journey is different for everyone. We aren't going to give you a specific to-do list, but we will teach you how to make your own. When you finish this book, you should know what you need to do, and how to get started on it. Knowing what your next three steps are will take a lot of the stress and uncertainty out of things.

We recommend that you start building a vet school binder where you can keep notes, create your master schedule for the next several years, and record your horse, work, volunteer, and veterinary experiences. Everything you do with jobs and horses matters, and you're going to need dates, names, phone numbers, and details on what you did. By the time you are ready to apply to vet school, you will have an extensive resume. That documented experience will be one of your most important assets. We've seen a lot of vet school application packets, and the ones with a long, clear history of horse, work, and veterinary experience really stand out. We'll talk more about this, too.

Keeping your perspective straight is important. There are a thousand things that happen between your freshman year in high school and your senior year in college. You don't have to be ready to handle every one of those things right now. You should have a broad understanding of the process, but don't try to do everything at once. Focus on the next three things on your list. When you accomplish those things, move on to the next three. You can handle three things! Eventually, you'll accomplish all one thousand things, three things at a time. Or two. Or one. It doesn't matter, as long as you find what works for you.

Keeping your perspective straight can also mean not listening to certain people. We call them *naysayers,* the people who tell you you're wasting your time, that you won't make it. Don't listen to them. They are usually secretly envious of you, and their own self-doubts get projected outward in an attack on people they think are better than them.

Sometimes these people are your friends, or even family members. That makes it harder to dismiss them, but you can't let them derail you. If it's someone you have to see every day, find a way to use their negativity as motivation to prove them wrong. You *can* do this.

We recommend that you begin a planned and focused path to vet school when you're a freshman in high school. If you're in sixth grade and you already know this is what you want to do, that's great! You can start now; you don't have to wait. The earlier you start gaining experience, the better.

Alright, let's get into it!

CHAPTER 1

BEING A PEOPLE PERSON

One thing we want to get right out front: At least 60% of being a veterinarian is dealing with people. Maybe even 70%. It is critical that you understand this concept. If you love animals, and you have a hard time being around people, you might think that becoming a veterinarian will be a great job for you. This is seldom the case!

Communicating with Clients

Equine veterinarians have to talk to horse owners all day, every day. They have to ask the right questions about what the horse is doing to get a clear understanding of the situation. Vets have to explain complicated medical things to owners in a way that they can understand, and teach them how to change bandages and apply eye medications. They have to explain their diagnosis and recommended treatment plan. Sometimes the owner can't afford to do what needs to be done, and the veterinarian has to work with them to find a solution. Sometimes that involves coming up with a different treatment plan. Sometimes it means euthanizing the horse.

Another tough thing veterinarians have to deal with all the time is collecting payments from clients. Having horses is expensive, and sometimes people can't pay the vet bill right away. That means you have to call them and ask for money. If they don't have it, you have to do it again next week. When people have a horse emergency, and don't have the money to pay you to come save their horse, you have to have a conversation with them about that. Having tough conversations with owners is part of being an equine veterinarian.

For general practitioners, the relationship they have with their clients is what keeps them in business. That means that even when it's a bad situation, the veterinarian has to be in control, and has to manage to situation and arrive at a solution that works for everyone. Sometimes what's right for the horse isn't what's right for the owner. Sometimes what's right for the owner isn't right for the veterinarian. This nearly always revolves around money. The owner can't or won't spend the money to do what the horse needs. The veterinarian can't work for free. The horse is stuck in the middle. As the veterinarian, you have to find the solution that allows you to do as much as you can for the horse, and maintain the relationship so you don't lose the client over it, and still cover your costs so you don't go out of business. This isn't an everyday occurrence, but it happens regularly, and you will need the skills to handle it.

Communicating with Staff

Managing staff is another big part of being a vet. This requires a lot of skills you won't necessarily get in vet school. As the veterinarian, you will be in charge of every situation. It's kind of like being the top cop at a crime scene. Everyone expects you to be in charge and have all the answers. The client expects you to manage the situation, and your technician or assistant does, too. If you have a vet student or a shadow riding along, you might have three or four people looking to you for direction and guidance.

If you have a technician or vet assistant, you'll often be teaching them how to do their job. This means everything from how to manage the horse while you do your job, to how to have a conversation with the client while you type up the bill and care instructions. That's right! Not only do you have to be a good communicator, you have to teach your team how to be good communicators, too. You'll end up teaching your tech a lot of things in front of the client, simply because of the circumstances. That means you have to be a good teacher, and you have to be able to do it under a bit of pressure from the audience.

Improving Your Communication Skills

As you are shadowing veterinarians, which we'll talk about extensively in another chapter, pay attention to all the conversations they have during the day. Try to picture yourself having those conversations. If the vet is doing it right, they are in charge in every conversation. That doesn't mean they are dominating the other person, quite the opposite. It means they are steering the discussion, making corrections when necessary, and arriving at the necessary point of conclusion. Sometimes that's easy, and sometimes it can be very difficult.

Pay attention to the difficult conversations and try to figure out how the veterinarian handled things right, and what they could have done better. Later, talk to the veterinarian about it. Ask them why they decided to handle it that way, what their thought process was. This is a great opportunity to learn about various factors that you might not know about, and increase your perspective.

Chances are, you aren't a world-class teacher and communicator. At least, not yet. Guess what? No one is a world-class teacher and communicator when they're 15. It's not something you're born with, it's a skill you develop over time. So, don't panic!

Like every other part of your journey to vet school, you can map out a plan to become an effective communicator and a good leader. Here are a few ways to do that:

- Seek out communications classes to increase your academic exposure

- Join clubs and volunteer for leadership positions

- Become a Teacher's Assistant

- Watch YouTube videos on leadership, teaching, and communication

- Read books! There are thousands of them on these topics

- Listen to podcasts. This is a free resource that can teach you a LOT about being a good leader

- Practice talking to people. Volunteer to work a booth at an event

- Give presentations to your classmates when you have the chance

With practice, you will get better and better at communicating. Be honest with yourself about your weak areas and focus on improving them. If you aren't sure what your weak areas are, ask someone you trust to give you some honest, critical feedback on your communication. Don't get your feelings hurt by what they say! Remember that you're asking for help, and they're trying to help you. Learning how others perceive you and your attempts to communicate is very important, and sometimes surprising!

Self-Awareness

Understanding your personality and tendencies is hugely helpful when you're trying to grow into something bigger and better. If you don't know where you're starting from, how can you get where you're going?

Taking a free online personality assessment is a great place to start. 16Personalities.com is a free Meyers-Briggs assessment tool that can tell you a lot. Just knowing whether you are an introvert or an extrovert is an important bit of knowledge. 5Voices.com is another great assessment tool, and their podcast, *GiANT's Liberator Podcast*, is a wonderful resource for understanding and learning to communicate with people who are a different personality type than you.

These assessments tell you how you function, what your processes are, your strengths and weaknesses, and your tendencies. Once you have a better understanding of yourself, you can identify the obstacles that you'll need to overcome to become a good communicator and a good leader. Don't worry, we all have these obstacles! Good leaders are aware of them and change their habits to get better, and bad leaders are oblivious to their own shortcomings.

Being self-aware, and demonstrating that on your vet school application, will make you a much stronger candidate. They aren't looking for someone who is perfect, they're looking for someone who is aware of their weaknesses and is actively working to improve. So, when it comes time to talk about that stuff, remember this! Don't be afraid to be honest. Consider the following two examples.

Example 1

> *My biggest fault is probably that I care too much. When I get really involved in something, I work really hard on it, and sometimes people say that I work too hard. Caring a lot and working hard are things that will make me a great veterinarian, so I guess it isn't all bad!*

Example 2

> *As an introvert, my natural tendency is to remain quiet and allow others to lead a conversation. This is not an ideal attribute for a veterinarian. To overcome this, I have taken a public speaking course*

to get more comfortable talking in front of others. I have also taken a leadership role in three different organizations to gain leadership experience and practice taking charge of discussions. While I'm not perfect yet, I'm a lot better than I was when I started, and I continue to work on this aspect of myself.

Example 1 uses a worn-out trope that every job interviewer has heard a thousand times: *I work too hard, I care too much.* This is an instant red flag response. It tells the interviewer or screener that you either don't have any self-awareness, or you're not being honest. Either way, that's a strike against you.

Example 2 shows that you know about this shortcoming, why it's a big deal, and what you're trying to do about it. This tells the interviewer that you are mature, growth-oriented, and willing to go the extra mile to achieve your goals.

Here's a real-world example from the authors of this book, Dr. Lacher and Justin Long. When she took the 5Voices assessment, Dr. Lacher discovered that her voice order was Creative, Pioneer, Connector, Guardian, Nurturer. You'll learn more about each of these voices from their website, books, and podcast, but here's a brief synopsis of what it means for Dr. Lacher.

Creative is her strongest voice. Creatives have lots of ideas, and love to try new things. They also tend to be unorganized, and don't always finish what they start. Each voice has strengths, but they also have weaknesses.

Pioneer is her second voice, and nearly as strong as her first. Pioneers are good at being in charge. They have lots of self-confidence and motivation, and they don't rely on other people's opinions. However, they also have a tendency to bulldoze their way through the world without realizing or worrying about how this affects those around them.

For Dr. Lacher, understanding these things about herself allows her to get a clearer look at her strengths and weaknesses. Knowing that she is naturally unorganized tells her that she needs a Guardian on her team. Guardians are very organized, and since she's running a business, organization is important.

Nurturer is her weakest voice, and Nurturers are good at managing personal relationships. Being weak in this area is a major liability for Dr. Lacher. As a veterinarian, building and maintaining good relationships with her clients and her staff will make a tremendous difference in the success of her veterinary clinic as well as her quality of life.

Dr. Lacher knows that she is naturally wired to jump from one thing to another, run over people without getting input from them, and not realize that she might have hurt someone's feelings. To overcome these obstacles, she focuses a lot of energy on creating processes that change her behavior. In staff meetings, she makes it a point to invite input from everyone on the team on a new idea. She checks in with the Nurturers and Connectors on her team, as they will always know how everyone feels about things. She lets most decisions that impact the team be made as a team decision, rather than handling it on her own. She takes time to think about things, rather than acting on instinct. Over time, these things have become habit, and she has effectively changed her behavior.

Justin, her husband, is a Nurturer, Guardian, Pioneer, Connector, Creative. He's sensitive and organized and is her opposite in many ways. His tendencies make him a great business partner for her, as well as a great life partner. His strengths cover her weaknesses, and her strengths cover his weaknesses. And because they're committed to self-awareness and personal growth, they understand each other better, not just themselves.

Fostering self-awareness in their veterinary clinic has helped them understand their team members, and their team members understand themselves and each other. This makes it a great place to work. When you understand the strengths and weaknesses of not only yourself, but those you work with, you don't create unrealistic expectations. You can also avoid setting yourself and others up to fail. How? By assigning people to tasks that they are suited for. Guardians are great with organization, and Creatives aren't. If you have a Creative doctor, she needs a Guardian technician to help her cover all the bases. Connectors are people-people, so they work well at answering the phone and interacting with your clients, as well as managing teams. Nurturers will make sure that everything gets done and keep everyone happy while they do it.

It takes all different kinds of people to make a great team, so no matter where you fall on the personality spectrum, you bring value. The important part is knowing what your strengths and weaknesses are, and actively working to improve yourself.

The earlier you identify things that you need to work on, the more time you'll have to work on them and build skills. These are also things that can go in your binder. You might have a whole list of things that you've worked on by the time you apply to vet school, and you don't want to forget any of them. When you're interviewing in-person, these things make great discussion topics, and the impression you make in that interview will decide your future.

CHAPTER 2

BUILDING YOUR BINDER

Everything we discuss in this book is about preparing you for vet school and going through the application and interview process. Experience is crucial, and documenting that experience is equally crucial. Your binder will be a living document where you keep track of everything you've done, and everything you need to do.

Some people are naturally organized, and others are naturally chaotic. If you are naturally chaotic, you will need to put measures into place to create organization in your life. Everything about being a doctor revolves around systems and processes, so learning to create those now will make it easier for you for the rest of your life. If you're naturally organized, give yourself a high five! Reading books like *The Checklist Manifesto* by Atul Gawande can help you create new habits and improve your ability to cover all the bases.

We recommend getting a 3-ring binder to keep everything together. Keep your pages in plastic sleeves to prevent them from getting torn or smudged. You'll need a few thumb drives, or memory sticks, too. Over the next few years, you will develop a collection of online documents that are important, and you can save them on your thumb drive and keep it in your binder. Always back everything up on a second thumb drive, just in case. A keyring is a great way to attach the thumb drive to your binder ring, so it doesn't get lost. Organization rule #1: Keep everything together!

If you are horrified by the idea of doing this with a physical binder, the same thing can be accomplished using a computer. If you choose this option, you need to use cloud-based storage, such as Google Docs, DropBox, or something similar. Having your digital binder on a computer or external hard drive is a very bad plan, as you can lose everything if it crashes. Remember, you'll be building and using this for ten years or more, and you'll go through several computers during that time. Protecting your data is paramount!

We're going to explain the binder as a physical 3-ring binder. If you decide to go digital, just apply the concepts in a digital way. Instead of sections, create folders. Label everything the same way, and label your individual documents clearly so you can tell what they are at a glance. As time goes by, you'll have a lot of files in there, so start organizing properly on day one.

Binder Layout

You can use dividers, or tabs, to break your binder into sections and keep everything organized. Organization! It starts here. It might seem like overkill in the beginning when you don't have much to put in it, but it will fill up, don't worry. This binder will be both your resume and your road map to vet school. You're going to have this binder from now until you finish vet school, and if you keep it organized right from the start, it will always be easy to use. The way you use it will change over time, and the information you put in it now will be what you have to refer back to later, so cover all your bases right from the start.

Here are some section titles that you'll need to put in your binder:

- All Equine Vets in My Area

- All Small Animal Vets in My Area

- Horse Experience (non-veterinary)

- Vets I've Shadowed

- Places I've Worked (non-veterinary)

- Places I've worked (veterinary)

- Places I've Volunteered

- Places I'd like to Work

- Places I'd like to Extern

- Places I'd like to Intern

- Social Awareness

- Self-improvement Activities

- Master Calendar

Each one of these sections will be a place to track your experience, or track what you need to do yet, and will need certain information depending on what it is. Let's look at a few sample page entries from a binder:

HORSE EXPERIENCE

Personal Horses: Owned two horses since I was 9. My parents taught me how to feed them, and I was responsible for feeding and cleaning stalls from ages 12-18. I assisted the farrier and the vet during all visits. Gave medications to horses as directed by vet, including IM shots and bandage changes. I did trail riding from ages 12-14, then switched to show jumping from age 14 - present. Took lessons with a trainer from ages 14 - present on a weekly basis.

Working Student: Cleaned and fed 18-stall barn on weekends from age 16-18. Hacked 6 horses most weekends, and groomed multiple horses for trainer at horse shows, 10 shows per year. Rode trainer's horses at shows for potential buyers.

Trainer: Wendy Brady (888) 555-1313

*Note: This section will probably be several pages of entries by the time you get to vet school. That's okay! Write everything down. You can decide what to include on your vet school application later.

Vets I've Shadowed

Vet Name: Dr. Marsha Brady
Practice: Mayberry Equine Veterinary Services
Location: Mayberry, IL
Practice phone: 888-555-1212
Practice email: MEVS@MEVS.com
Dates: July 2020 - August 2020
Number of weeks: 6
Hours per week: 20

Experiences: helped administer core vaccines, assisted in ultrasounding lower limbs during lameness eval, observed artificial insemination on 3 different mares, observed 6 dental floats, observed diagnosis and treatment of a gas colic, observed eye ulcer through ophthalmoscope and administered eye meds via subpalpebral lavage multiple times, attended a euthenasia.

Note to self: Great hands-on! I liked Dr. Brady, would be happy to work here later on.

*Note: Make sure you add the places you want to return to as an employee, extern, or intern to the appropriate page in your binder.

Places I've Worked (non-veterinary)

Outback Steakhouse
May 2019 - October 2019
Position: Server
Hours per week: 30
Phone: (877) 333-2211

Duties: Take food orders, refill drinks, provide great customer service with a smile!

Pizza Hut
Jan 2019 - May 2019
Position: Delivery driver

Hours per week - 18
Phone: (877) 333-2233

Duties: Driving, delivering pizza, customer service, dispute resolution.

Hall County SPCA
April 2018 - December 2018
Position: Public Outreach
Hours per week: 16

Duties: fundraising events, create public awareness campaigns, organize adoption events, coordinate volunteers for events.

*Note: This section might have 2 employers, or it might have 10. That's okay! Write them all down, and be detailed about your duties. You'd be surprised at what translates into useful skills to the admissions committee. Just because it seems irrelevant to you now doesn't mean you shouldn't write it down.

Places I've Volunteered

Name: Mayberry Horse Rescue
Location: Mayberry, IL
Phone: 888-555-1414
Dates: Jan 2018- August 2020
Number of weeks: 45

Hours per week: 6 (1 Saturday per month during school year)

Duties: Groomed horses, mucked paddocks, assisted veterinarian during exams as needed, unloaded hay, gave tours to visitors.

Name: Hall County SPCA
Location: Mayberry, IL
Phone: (877) 333-2211
Dates: August 2020 - Dec 2020
Number of weeks: 18
Hours per week: 8

Duties: Cleaned kennels, groomed animals for adoption events, walked dogs, play time/socialization time with animals.

Note to self: I do not want to be an extern here! Zero hands-on time, and not a learning environment AT ALL. The externs don't even get to assist the vet with spays and neuters.

It's a good idea to write down interesting events that happen in the places you work or volunteer, even if they don't have anything to do with veterinary medicine. These things can make for good side discussions in interviews, and writing them down will help you build a journal of sorts that you can reflect back on before an interview. If you accumulate enough of these, you might even create a section in your binder just for them.

MASTER CALENDAR

The calendar section can get complicated, and you might find that you need a variety of timeline tools to keep track of everything. Digital calendars with reminders, such as Google Calendar, are a great tool, so don't hesitate to integrate technology into your system.

Once you've identified all the equine veterinarians in your area, you'll want to start working on a shadowing schedule. When you first start, you'll likely only be able to schedule one ride-along with each vet. Once you've done that ride-along and proved yourself to be a worthy shadow (we'll talk all about that in the shadowing section), then you'll have the opportunity to schedule future shadowing dates. If you're diligent, you will get your next six months, or a year of shadowing lined up. The earlier you are on the schedule, the less trouble you'll have competing for time slots with other shadows.

Another way your Master Calendar is useful is getting your timeline down in a way that you can see it and make sense of it. You will have various things that you need to start and finish by certain times, and you can list those things out, so you know what's coming up that you need to prepare for. This includes things like scholarship applications, college applications, requesting letters of recommendation, and so on. It can also be a way to track goals. For example, you might decide you want to shadow four veterinarians each year. As the year is winding down, you'll need a reminder to schedule your next few shadowing opportunities. As you accomplish these things, you can look back over your calendar and see how much you've done.

One way of creating a master calendar is printing a blank monthly calendar with big squares that you can write in, like this:

Sunday	Monday	Tuesday	Wednesday	Thursday	Friday	Saturday

You can find these blank calendars for free on the internet and print more as you need them.

Using your Binder

As you start shadowing veterinarians, you can start filling in some of the other sections in your binder. It might seem like it's unnecessary to write everything down at first, but as you accumulate more and more data, it will become too much to remember. So, once you've started shadowing a vet, write down your start date, all the contact information, and start a list of what you've watched and done. Once you've been there enough to know if it would be a good place to extern or work, you can add it to your list in those sections. By the time you get close to graduating high school, you should have a thorough list of places you'd like to work over the summer. If you did a good job as a shadow, then you already have a good relationship with them, and that makes lining up a summer job far easier.

When you get to college, there will be more demands on your time. You should continue to accumulate animal experience, but the number of places you do that will probably drop. That's okay! Your binder will continue to fill up as your experience grows. You will also likely have some new opportunities to add to it. If your college has an agricultural department, you might be able to work as a lab assistant and get poultry, swine, or cattle experience. Not only will this broaden your skills, it might even expose you to career opportunities that you didn't know existed. If nothing else, it will make you a more well-rounded candidate for vet school, and that's important.

One of the nice things about shadowing with a lot of veterinarians is that you can start building a collection of letters of reference for future job applications. You won't want to ask for one if you haven't spent much time there, but for the places you go a lot and have built a relationship with, it's certainly appropriate to ask them for a general letter of recommendation for jobs, externships, and internships.

Later on, you'll need some veterinarians to write you a recommendation letter for vet school, so building those relationships is important. We see a lot of recommendation letters, and when they come from someone you've shadowed for a long time as well as worked for, that counts for a lot more than a professor who had you for one class. If you do a good job with your binder, you'll know exactly who to ask and how to reach them.

Tracking dates and names, along with contact information, is one of the primary functions of your binder. If you've shadowed twelve veterinarians and had four jobs over the last eight years, the only way you'll be able to accurately fill out the *Experience* portion of your vet school application is if you took good notes along the way. Your vet school application is going to request all of the information we've listed for you to track, and it's very important to have it.

CHAPTER 3

HORSE EXPERIENCE

Are you a horse person? If you're not, you need to work on becoming one. Vet school will teach you how horses work on the inside, but that's only half of it. You need to know how horses eat, think, react, and move. You need to know their tics and quirks. You need to be comfortable handling them, touching them, and guiding them to move in particular ways, and recognizing when they can't. Maybe most important, you need to speak the language. Communicating with horse owners is a huge part of being a horse vet, and if you don't speak their language, you'll be at a huge disadvantage.

Riding Experience

Having experience riding horses, regardless of the discipline, will teach you a lot of things you need to know. Working with a trainer is very beneficial, as they'll teach you many things you might never figure out on your own.

Whether you're into western pleasure, hunter/jumpers, barrel racing, or dressage, learning a discipline will help you learn horses and horse people in a way that nothing else will. It will also keep you around horse people and talking about horses, and every bit of that helps.

If you end up becoming a general practitioner, or a specialist who works with sport horses and lameness issues, having a good understanding of several popular disciplines will be to your advantage. You don't necessarily need to train in every discipline, but you should spend some time getting to know each one, and consider training in at least two different disciplines. When you are talking to your clients about their horses, and what they are trying to accomplish, you will have much more success if you know what they're talking about. Think about it this way: if you ride dressage, and your horse is having trouble with the half pass, who do you want to talk to about it? A veterinarian who knows exactly what you're talking about, or a veterinarian who doesn't know what a half pass is?

While lessons from horse trainers usually cost money, there are other ways to learn if you can't afford to pay for it. Working for a horse trainer is a great way to learn. While you're taking care of the horses and keeping the barn clean, you're earning lessons. And when you get good enough, trainers that have a lot of horses to be worked will put you to work riding horses. You can learn a lot about horses from riding three or four different horses on a regular basis, so becoming a working student is a great way to bolster your horse knowledge. Even if money isn't an issue, this is a great way to gain riding experience.

Ground Handling Skills

The other half of horse experience is learning to handle horses from the ground. While riding will help you communicate with horse people, learning groundwork will help you communicate with the horse. There are a variety of styles of groundwork, and we recommend that you learn one of them now, as that will make everything you do going forward more effective. Horses are big, heavy animals, and they can hurt you. That means you need to know how to manage them while you're working on them, and you also need to be able to train those who are working with you to handle them properly, for your safety as well as theirs. The more you understand horse behavior, the better you'll become at anticipating their actions under specific circumstances.

Basic horse training skills, such as clicker training, can be a huge advantage for a veterinarian. Whether you're working with a needle-shy horse, or one that won't load on the trailer, having the skill to quickly change the horse's behavior will make you more efficient, improve the safety of you and your team, and increase the confidence of the client. You can learn a lot of these concepts with free videos on YouTube, and practice them on your horse, or other horses in your barn. As with all skills, the more you do it, the better you'll get.

Variety is the Spice of Life

If all of your horse experience so far has been with one or two breeds, you should try to spend some time around horses of different breeds. Quarter horses have a very different temperament than Arabs or warmbloods. Ponies, donkeys, and minis all have their own characteristics. Draft horses are as different from thoroughbreds as they could be. As a veterinarian, you are likely to encounter a wide variety of breeds every day, and you'll need to know how they differ from one another.

If you're already a horse person, and have grown up riding, that's great! You're ahead of the game. Don't stop now! If you haven't done much groundwork, we urge you to add that into your regimen. The more well-rounded your horse skills, the better everything will go for you. If you are well-experienced in riding and groundwork, then you are doing all the right things. Keep it up, and work on diversifying your breed and discipline experience.

Every minute you spend with a horse, whether it's yours or at a barn where you work or ride, pay attention to everything. Practice paying attention to his breathing, heart rate, attitude, mannerisms, and movements. Eventually this will become a habit, and this is a habit you want to foster and grow. When you are highly attuned to normal, healthy horses, it will be easier for you to pick up on signs that something is wrong.

While horse rescues don't typically have a veterinarian on staff, they often have horses who are in a rehab situation, and you can gain experience working with them. Don't forget, if you are a working student at a training barn, that counts as animal experience! If you grew up mucking stalls and taking care of your horse, that counts, too. It tells the admissions committee that you know horses, and this isn't something you got excited about two months ago. They want to see that you have done your homework, and you know by a lot of experience that this is what you want to do with your life.

Gaining valuable horse experience

If you need more horse experience, and you probably do, here are a few places and ways you can find it:

- Training barns - either as a paying student or as a working student, employee, or volunteer

- Horse Rescues - they all need volunteers

- Horse shows - as an employee or volunteer, or even as a spectator

- Seminars - some equine clinics offer free seminars

- Clinics - trainers of all kinds host clinics all over the country

- 4H, Pony Club, and other riding organizations for young people

- Horse camps, either as a rider or a volunteer

CHAPTER 4

HIGH SCHOOL

Remember when we were talking about developing time management skills? It starts now. Having a part-time job in high school, riding with your trainer, shadowing an equine vet, maintaining your grades, and doing some extra-curricular activities in school will require you to get really good at managing your time.

Working

One good way to do this is to combine some of those things. If you can get a job at a barn, whether it's with your trainer or somewhere else, you can continue to build your horse experience and groundwork skills while learning how to juggle all the things. Many kids arrive at college with no time management skills, and their freshman grades reflect that. Poor grades can hurt your application packet, so having experience at managing all those things before you get to college will put you ahead of many others who are competing for those coveted seats in vet school.

If having a horse, or hiring a trainer is a financial challenge for you and your family, becoming a working student at a horse farm is a great way to accomplish several goals at once. Many trainers will give you lessons in exchange for labor. Mucking stalls, grooming horses, and even riding them for the trainer are activities that you can do. This will give you work experience, horse experience, and life experience in terms of finding a way to finance your dreams.

If you have the horse experience covered and you're more interested in getting some other kind of job, doing anything that is customer service-oriented will give you valuable skills. Why is that important? Because vet school might teach you how to diagnose and treat the problem with the horse, but handling a stressed-out owner is all up to you. These people are your customers, your clients, and you want them to continue to be your clients. That means you have to manage your relationship with them in both good times and bad. When it comes to people's horses, the bad times can be bad. The more time you've spent waiting tables in a restaurant, or answering phones at a veterinary clinic, the better prepared you will be to handle things appropriately and professionally.

Another benefit to working in high school is that you get

accustomed to making and managing money. Everyone does this badly in the beginning, and that's okay. If you're still living at home, you have a safety net while you learn to manage your budget. When you get to college, it's much more complicated to avoid spending more than you have to live on. By the time you get to vet school, you need to be a rock-solid money manager. If you aren't, your student loans will become unmanageable. One of the biggest problems young veterinarians face today is staggering student loan debt. You can avoid some of that by being money-smart before you start.

If you have a financial benefactor that will be helping you pay for college, you can use the money you earn from working to live on or save it to live on during vet school.

Shadowing

This is one of the most important things you can do for yourself. Like many professions, being a veterinarian involves a whole lot of things that you don't realize until you either become one, or spend a lot of time with one. Most veterinarians are happy to let you ride along with them and see what it's really like, and this is called shadowing the veterinarian.

You should do this with several different veterinarians, and not just once or twice. The goal here is that you find out whether this is really what you want to do *before* you spend all the time and money to become a veterinarian. Finding out in vet school, or even after you graduate, that you don't actually like doing this is a tragedy, and it's completely avoidable. And yet, it happens.

This is the first step in intense familiarization with veterinary medicine. It will be hard to mesh your schedule with a vet during the school year, but spring break, summer break, and long holiday weekends are great times to make this happen. Depending on where you live, there might be some logistical challenges to overcome, so do your homework ahead of time. Find out which equine veterinarians in your area allow shadowing and ask them what their policies are. Find out what days they do this, how far in advance you need to sign up, and what you should bring with you. Some veterinarians get lots of shadows, and you might be on a long waiting list. With many equine vets, this will be an all-day experience. You may need to bring all your food and drinks for the day.

Sometimes you'll leave at 8:00 am and won't get back until 6:30 or 7:00 pm, or later. In equine general practice, you spend a lot of time going from one farm to another, and if an emergency calls, that can throw a wrench in the schedule. This is great experience for you as a high school student, as you'll get to see what it's really like. You need to make sure your parents understand the situation, so they don't freak out if you're gone all day long and don't make it back for supper.

Some high schools have programs that allow students to do things like this on school days. Check with your school to see if that's an option. If you can shadow a vet every other Friday, go for it! Just make sure that your academics don't suffer as a result of it. That's not a good trade.

Once you're out of high school, we're going to urge you to get a job with a veterinarian as an assistant, technician, or something along those lines. While you're shadowing as many vets as you can in high school, pay attention! This is your opportunity to shop all the places around that you might want to work in a few years. This is a solid gold opportunity to try them all out first. Who else gets to do that? Keep good notes on who is a good teacher, who lets you get hands on with things, who you *don't* want to work for, and so on.

In addition to shadowing horse vets, you can also shadow small animal vets, cattle vets, chicken vets, marine vets, or wildlife vets. All veterinary experience counts on your vet school application, and having a well-rounded set of experiences will show that you are familiar with a broad spectrum of animal medicine. There's no such thing as having too much experience.

If you live near a vet school, you can get some great experience shadowing doctors and technicians there. Large equine referral hospitals are also a great place to gain some perspective and experience. Depending on where you live, you might have to travel a bit to get to a referral hospital, but the experience you'll get at a place like that is fantastic.

Many vet schools have a Pre-Vet Advisor. This person's job is to help you get prepared for vet school, and they will start working with you in high school or college to help you get on track and make sure you're covering all the bases. Some vet schools even offer vet camps, where you can come spend a week at the vet school and learn more about it. This is a great opportunity to begin building a relationship with a vet school, as well as some veterinary professionals.

We'll talk much more about shadowing in the next chapter, so don't worry if you still have questions!

Classes

Becoming a veterinarian requires a lot of science classes, of course, but it's important to realize how important your English and math classes are, as well. You have to use math to calculate the weight of a horse using a weight tape. Once you know the horse weighs 1,200 pounds, you have to calculate the proper dose of the drug he needs. The drug instructions say to administer 3mgs per kg. Whoa, what? That's right, now you have to figure out how many kilograms are in 1,200 pounds, and then how many milligrams of the drug to give. The syringe is labeled in cc's, not mg's. It can get complicated. You also need to be able to look over a bill and make sure it's correct. If you are a solo practitioner, you might even be doing your own bookkeeping. You definitely need to know how to keep the books straight!

Another critical part of math is understanding how loans work. Unless you have a very wealthy benefactor who is paying for your college and graduate school, you are looking at some very large student loans. It's hard to make sense of what it means to be $300,000 in debt, especially when you haven't even made it to the point of being financially independent. We're going to talk about student loans later in the book to help you with this, but for now, we'll say that people who understand money and loans are far less likely to be taken advantage of or find themselves in a bad situation.

English classes are important, too. If you're going to maintain a high GPA throughout high school and college, you're going to write a million papers, and they need to be well written. You're also going to spend a great deal of your career writing emails to potential employers, vendors, and clients. If you work in a lab or at a vet school, you might even contribute to or author research papers that get published. If your writing skills are poor, people will assume your veterinary skills are poor too, even if you're a great vet. That can keep you from being successful.

The same goes for speaking ability. You are the translator for your clients, as most of them don't speak doctor. They might be impressed by all the big words you know, but if they don't know what you're talking about, then you are doing them a disservice. You need to be an effective communicator, and that means speaking in terms people can clearly understand without sounding demeaning or condescending, and still explaining everything they need to know to make a decision about their horse. It might sound easy, but it isn't. Being an effective communicator is a skill, and skills are developed.

One way you can start developing your communication skills is to seek out opportunities to make presentations to your class. This will help you get comfortable speaking in front of others, which is another important skill, and it will also help you learn how to gauge your audience and know if you are connecting with them or not. In addition to your English classes, you can seek out videos on YouTube to enhance your public speaking skills.

Advanced Placement, IB, or dual-enrollment classes are common at many high schools. These programs allow high school students to take college courses, giving them college credits, or even an associate's degree upon completion of high school. Nearly everyone we talked to while researching this book took AP classes, and nearly all of them said they were glad they did. Some took dual enrollment classes as well. Some were glad they did, some didn't get what they had hoped from them.

While this is a positive experience for many students, there are some things you need to research and consider. The most important of these is the college you plan to go to for your undergraduate degree. Not all colleges and universities recognize dual enrollment credits. Some students arrive at college thinking they're on track to have a bachelor's degree in two years, and find out their college doesn't recognize their credits. This is not the time to figure this out!

We'll talk more about colleges in the next chapter, but before you start taking AP or dual enrollment classes, find out which colleges recognize them, and which don't. If the big-name school you like doesn't recognize them, you might be better off going to a different college. Some smaller universities and community colleges have excellent degree programs that will recognize your credits and still get you ready for vet school. They can be significantly cheaper, too, and that will be a big deal for you in the long run. If you're committed to a college that doesn't recognize these credits, then use your time in high school to gain other relevant experiences instead of taking extra classes.

Time Management

Being super-busy in high school is a great way to learn how to manage your time. If you drop the ball, and you probably will, the consequences are less dire than they will be later on in college and vet school. So, this is the time to figure it out.

Everyone has different needs when it comes to allocating study time and sleep time. As you are juggling school, extra-curricular activities, homework, AP classes, riding horses, shadowing vets, volunteering, and working, you are probably going to find yourself over-extended. You'll have to cut something out of your schedule or re-prioritize so that you don't drop everything. This is an important process, as you need to know how far you can go, and how far is too far.

Creating strong boundaries now will keep you from over-extending in college, which is a mistake many people make. Students who sailed through high school with minimal studying often don't allot enough time for studying when they get to college, and as their first semester comes to a close, they realize they'll have to drop a class to avoid failing it. College is different from high school. The classes are harder and more varied, and if you have too many demands on your time, you can get in trouble. Getting a D in Organic Chemistry can definitely haunt you later, so don't wait until you get to college to learn how you function best.

Stress Management Tools

Along with a packed schedule and high expectations for yourself comes stress. Like

managing your time, managing your stress is another skill that is best developed early. Nearly every vet student and veterinarian we spoke to said the same thing: develop tools for stress early on. For many of them, a regular exercise program worked great. It's a proven fact that keeping your body fit will improve your mood and attitude. Active sports are also useful, as they involve camaraderie with teammates as well as physical activity.

If exercise and sports are not your thing, it's important to figure out what is. Reading, writing, music, and art are also popular engagements. While they're lacking the endorphin rush of exercise, they do involve a high level of creative brain power, which is very satisfying. If you don't have a preferred stress management routine yet, now is the time to start experimenting. Many people find swimming, yoga, mindfulness meditation, or dance to be useful too, or even martial arts classes.

Once you find what works for you, make it a regular part of your daily or weekly routine. Stress management tools only work if you use them, so don't rely on something that you don't use regularly, like kayaking or surfing. While those things certainly have their place, you need something you can do without it being a special occasion.

Don't Forget to Have Fun!

High school is a crazy time in life. Don't get so caught up in trying to do all the things that you forget to enjoy yourself! Do social things, make time to hang out with your friends, go to horse shows, do whatever it is that you do. Life is meant to be lived!

CHAPTER 5

SHADOWING A VETERINARIAN

Shadowing is a term we use for people who follow a veterinarian around to see what all they do. This is also called "volunteering," but we're going to refer to it only as shadowing. Volunteering is another thing that you'll be doing, and we don't want to get the two confused. So, for the purposes of this book: if you're observing a veterinarian for a day, that's shadowing. If you're working in a soup kitchen, that's volunteering. If you're volunteering at an animal shelter, then it depends on what you're doing as to whether you're shadowing or volunteering. Make sense?

Hands-On Experience

As a shadow, you might not get much hands-on time. That's okay! You can still learn a lot by watching. One thing you should pay attention to is the other people there. Is there a technician who is trying to get into vet school? How much time does the vet spend teaching them? Do they get hands-on experience? This is important, because you might be that technician in a few years. Keep notes in your binder about which veterinarians are good teachers. When it comes time to look for a job, you'll already know where you want to work.

Small Animal Clinics

Wait, how is this helpful experience? In many ways! For starters, there are probably ten small animal clinics for every equine veterinarian in your region, if not more. If there are five other kids trying to shadow equine vets, then competition is fierce for the time slots available. While you want to get as much equine experience as possible, augmenting that with small animal experience will still be beneficial to you.

There are a lot of things that are the same across veterinary medicine that you can learn in a small animal clinic. Language, techniques, systems, and that sort of thing often cross-apply. You can learn about needles, catheters, forceps, and clamps. You can learn how to check heart rates, breathing rates, and symptoms of illness. You can learn how to take a patient history and order a blood test. You can answer phones, learn how to talk to clients, and make appointments. Getting to know the computer software can be hugely beneficial, especially if you learn more than one.

Another great advantage to spending some time in small animal clinics is the opportunity to see teams in action. If you watch carefully, you'll see how bad teams can disrupt the workflow in a clinic and create a toxic environment. Sometimes just one or two people can be at the root of it, but their negativity can suck everyone else down, too. These are important lessons to learn, because someday you will have your own team, and you need to be able to recognize when someone on your team is making it toxic.

If you're lucky, you'll also get to see some really good teams in action. Small animal clinics usually have more people than large animal clinics, unless you're at a big equine hospital. The more people there are on a team, the harder it is to keep everyone working together. Watch the good teams as well as the bad ones and try to learn what makes the good ones good, and the bad ones bad. Listen to the way the staff talks about the doctors, and vice versa. Watch how they interact with one another. Is there animosity? Respect? Do they work well together? How do they communicate with each other?

Teams are one of the most important parts of a veterinary clinic of any kind, but not all veterinary clinics focus on developing their teams to be high performers.

The better you understand teams, both good and bad, the better you'll be at being on a team, as well as managing one. Your team will have a massive impact on your quality of life, so don't take this lightly.

Another thing you can learn at small animal clinics is how to run a business. If you think you might want to own your own practice someday, or be a partner in a practice, there is a lot to learn that has nothing to do with being a veterinarian. Spending time with the practice manager and others on the business side of things will expose you to the processes that make everything work. Ordering drugs and supplies, relationships with vendor representatives, processing payroll, paying bills, bookkeeping, daily reports, managing staff issues, all of these things are part of making a clinic function, large or small.

If you own your own practice, you can hire people to do these things for you, right? Of course you can, and you should. As a doctor, your time is best spent doing doctor things. However, if you don't know how to do the business stuff, you won't know whether your team is doing a good job or robbing you blind. Unfortunately, veterinarians get robbed blind by their bookkeepers all the time. Once again, arming yourself with knowledge and experience now can save you endless problems later, and knowing every aspect of the business is important.

Small Equine Practices

Many equine veterinarians are solo practitioners, which means they work alone. Some of them have a tech, some of them have a receptionist who answers the phone and makes appointments, and some of them don't have anyone at all. Most of these work out of their truck, and don't have an office or a clinic.

Slightly larger small practices will have two or three veterinarians. Most of their work is still ambulatory, which means they go to wherever the horse is. Some of them will have a clinic, and some won't.

Riding along with these veterinarians is a fantastic way to see what life is like for a general practitioner. Their days can vary wildly. One appointment might be giving vaccines and doing a dental float, and the next one might be doing a lameness evaluation or ultrasounding a pregnant mare. You'll get to experience life on a small team and see how communication with clients works (or doesn't work). For many high school and college students, this can be the experience that tells you whether or not you want to continue your trek towards vet school, or perhaps look at some other career options.

One thing to consider before signing up to shadow an ambulatory veterinarian is that it might just be the two of you riding around together all day. Make sure that you meet them before committing yourself, and if you're in high school, maybe even have a parent come meet them with you. It's important to be comfortable with the person you're riding with, and always keep your personal safety as a priority.

Large Equine Practices

Big referral hospitals are very different from small equine practices. While they often see horses for wellness visits or lameness workups, they also perform surgeries, and that's a whole different world. Some people observe a surgery and decide they want nothing to do with that. Others observe a surgery and decide that's *exactly* what they want to do!

If you have an opportunity to shadow at a large equine practice, we highly recommend that you take it. However, it's important to understand how they function so that you have appropriate expectations for your experience there.

Most hospitals have an internship program. Veterinarians who just graduated from vet school will go work for these hospitals for a year as an intern, and that's how they really learn how to be a veterinarian and get a lot of experience. This will be on your to-do list for later on. These hospitals also have an extern program, in which students who are currently in vet school can come in for a few weeks at a time and get experience. Often some of the techs and nurses who work there are gaining experience while trying to get into vet school.

What does this mean for you? It means that as a shadow, you will get to observe, but you are at the bottom of the priority list for gaining experience. The interns are at the top of the list, and then the externs, and then the shadows. You'll get to see a lot of really cool things, but you probably won't get to actually do anything other than watch. That doesn't mean it's a wasted experience! You can still learn a ton of stuff, just know that it will all be by watching.

General Tips for getting the Best Experience

There are a lot of things that you can do to be a great shadow, and veterinarians will be happy to have you around and teach you everything you want to know. On the flip side of that, there are a lot of things you can do that will get you banned from shadowing someone, and you definitely want to avoid that. Here's a Do's and Don'ts list:

DO

- Be on time!

- Be engaged! Ask questions, answer questions, be part of the team

- Be willing to jump in and get your hands dirty

- Ask permission to try something, or handle an animal

- Respect the pecking order if there are others there for experience

- Take every opportunity to try something. If the vet asks if you want to do it, your answer should always be "Yes, please!"

- Pick up a broom and sweep. Unless you are actively sweeping where work is happening, this is never a wrong answer! If you show your willingness to work, you'll get a lot more opportunities to learn.

DON'T

- Be late

- Sleep at the clinic or in the vet truck

- Act unprofessional in front of a client

- Play on your phone

- Be a lump on a log

- Turn down opportunities to get hands-on

- No call/no show

- Disrespect the other staff members

Things you need to see before you apply for Vet School

Veterinarians do loads of different things. For many horse owners, all they've ever seen the veterinarian do is give vaccines, float their horse's teeth, and maybe do a pre-purchase exam or shoot radiographs for the farrier. This covers about 2% of what veterinarians actually do, and before you get to vet school, you need to participate in as many of those different things as you can. That way you have a clear picture of what being a veterinarian is all about, and if it's the right job for you. Here are some of the things that you need to see, and the earlier and more often you see them, the better:

Euthanasia: This is a big part of being a veterinarian. It's the veterinarian's responsibility to recognize when a horse needs to be euthanized, explain it to the owner, and then perform it. It's one thing to understand this on a philosophical level. It's another thing to actually do it. Make sure you attend a few of these events to confirm that you can handle it.

Blood and Guts: There are a variety of things that can happen to expose you to some pretty gory events. Lacerations, surgeries, injuries, all kinds of things. Make sure you can handle the blood and guts. Ask if you can glove up and help so you get a chance to touch things. If you explain your reason, you'll often get permission.

Foals being born: This might sound benign, but it really grosses some people out. When a foal is born, the vet needs to inspect the amniotic sac and placenta. That means picking it up, getting slime on you, and all that stuff. Make sure you're good with it by getting hands-on every chance you get.

Surgery: Watching surgeries is important. Not only is it the blood and guts factor, it's also the tenacity factor. Sometimes procedures can take a long time, and the vet is rarely in a comfortable position. When you're observing a surgery, pay attention to what the vet is going through. It's a big deal.

Difficult Conversations: You really need to see some vets having painful conversations with clients. Clients often cry during these events, or get angry, or both. Remember, it's a very big deal for them, especially if they don't have the money to do what they need to do, and the vet has to guide them through it. These interactions are really hard, because they're really important.

If you've found something that you can't handle, congratulations! Self-discovery is incredibly important. The more you know about yourself, the better you can make quality decisions regarding your future.

Also, don't panic! It doesn't necessarily mean you shouldn't be a veterinarian. It might, but then again, it might not. Talk to a vet about the thing you're worried about and ask their opinion on it. There are many things that you can do as a veterinarian aside from being a general practitioner or working in a referral hospital as a surgeon or an internal medicine veterinarian. See the chapter on alternative career paths for more on this topic.

Finding a Mentor

Finding a veterinarian to be your mentor will be a great benefit to you. As you start shadowing various vets in your area, you will probably find one that you really click with. Take advantage of this and build a relationship with that person!

Once you have a mentor, that doesn't mean that you stop shadowing other vets. It just means that you have a trusted guide and a dedicated resource. A mentor can answer lots of questions that you might not feel comfortable asking someone else. They're also more likely to take you under their wing and give you all the experiences they can, as opposed to just allowing you to observe.

A mentor isn't necessarily a friend. They can be a friend, but they also need to be willing to tell it to you straight and be honest with you when you're veering off course. Don't be afraid to be vulnerable with your mentor. They know you're not perfect, so if you can be honest about what you need help with, they can help you improve your weaknesses.

As you get closer to applying for vet school, your mentor will become an invaluable resource. Ask them to do practice interviews with you, and help you get stronger with your answers. When you write your essays for your vet school application, have them look over your work and give you feedback on it. They've been through the process and can keep you from making a mistake that no one else would even catch. You can also do practice job interviews with them. Use their experience to prepare yourself as much as possible.

There's nothing wrong with having more than one mentor. Some people have a certain professor that they click with, as well as a veterinarian. Having a mentor in the different areas of your life can be helpful. As with all things, don't overdo it. Too many cooks spoil the stew, as the saying goes. If you find your mentors giving you conflicting advice on important things, consider backing away from one slightly, and try to keep perspective on who has the best understanding of your trajectory.

CHAPTER 6

COLLEGE

Picking a College

You may be tempted to pick the college closest to you with a veterinary school. That's reasonable! Be sure it's the right choice for you. Starting at a smaller college has many benefits. One big advantage is more one-on-one time with professors. In general, it is easier to access helpful resources at smaller colleges. Look at finances. Veterinary school will require significant financial resources. Saving money by attending a college near home, or the one that offers you the best scholarships is far more important than attending a college with an affiliated vet school.

The number one thing to do once you are in college is to enjoy the experience! Many people are in a rush to get through as fast as they can. Taking longer to complete your undergraduate education isn't bad as long as you show you can handle the rigors of vet school. For example, don't take 8 credit hours each semester with an extracurricular activity load of 3 hours per week, and no job. Eight credit hours with significant hours employed, and some volunteer hours shows you have good time management skills and can handle the stress of a packed schedule. Be sure you demonstrate your ability to handle a serious time crunch at some point in your college career. It is important to keep a solid GPA, but a 4.0 is far from necessary. The core science classes like chemistry and biology do carry more weight, so put all your efforts into those classes.

We'll talk a lot more about the cost of your education in the chapter on student loans, but it's important to understand how significant that cost is. This needs to be a factor when you're looking at your undergrad options. Unless you have a wealthy benefactor, who will be paying all your education costs, and maybe even if you do, it's important to consider how the money you borrow today will impact your life down the road.

As we talked about in the chapter on high school, making sure any credits from high school are recognized by the colleges you're applying to is important. If you graduated high school with an AA degree, then you might only need to go to college for two years instead of four, so you want to make sure it's going to work before you commit. Paying for two years of tuition with scholarships is much more achievable than four years for many people, and if you can get through undergrad with little or no student loan debt, that will help you out tremendously.

Another option many people find best is going to a community or city college for the first two years, and then transferring to a bigger school for the rest of undergrad. This will cut your costs significantly. It's also a smoother transition from the pace of high school to the pace of college. Just like checking on your dual enrollment credits, make sure that the community or city college credits are recognized by the school you intend to transfer to. In particular, look into the required classes for veterinary school, such as organic chemistry and physics, and see if the vet schools you are interested in require that these classes be taken at a 4 year college. If so, just take the prerequisites and other courses not required for vet school at the community college.

Majors

You will experience serious pressure to figure this out early in your college career. Resist this pressure. Take this opportunity to explore a variety of options available at your college. Be sure you are taking the basics, like chemistry and biology, but also explore psychology, sociology, music, whatever intrigues you. That will help you know that you've picked the right career path. All knowledge is related, and you never know when that seemingly-unrelated class will apply to veterinary medicine.

Work to find a major that you enjoy, and that offers job opportunities beyond veterinary school. This will give you greater flexibility if you decide veterinary medicine isn't the career for you. You don't even have to major in biology or other core science majors. As long as all the prerequisites for veterinary school are completed, you can major in anything you want!

If you think that owning your own practice is something you might want to do someday, taking business classes is a good idea. Some veterinarians even have an entrepreneurial or business degree to help them be successful business owners. Others focus on psychology and communication, which helps them connect with their clients and staff, as well as market their practice to their community.

A lot of students choose to get a degree in animal sciences, as it seems like a good pre-vet track. While there are some benefits to this major, it also has some drawbacks. First and foremost, while you're in college, you may discover that you don't actually want to be a veterinarian after all. If it's not the career for you, and you realize that during your junior year of college, then you're ¾ of the way through a degree that won't help you out with whatever it is that you end up doing.

Many majors will benefit you as a veterinarian, but will also allow you to do a variety of other things. Some people fall in love with research in college, or teaching. College will expose you to many career possibilities that you may not even know exist, so even if you're pretty sure you won't change your mind, it's a good idea to avoid painting yourself into a corner.

Get a job in college

This is so very important! While it can be difficult to get a veterinary job, any job in a service industry will give you valuable experience when it comes to client interaction. Having a job also teaches you important people skills. You will learn how to work in teams, and what kind of environment you work best, and worst in. Getting a job to earn money is great, but it comes with many, many other valuable lessons you will use in your future career.

You should have had a job or two in high school, and by the time you get to college, you should have a decent understanding of how things work in a business. As someone who may very well own their own business someday, you should treat every job you have like a lab. Observe, collect data, and learn. Learn what makes things work, learn what makes things *not* work. Learn how people behave at work. Learn what makes the manager a good manager, or a bad manager. Learn what makes customers like the business or hate the business.

Think about what you would do if it was your business.

Experiences

There are many opportunities presented to you in college. For example, many colleges have study-abroad programs. These can be a great way to visit faraway places with a safety net in place. Many of these programs also offer a way to guarantee some experiences. If you are going to a South African veterinary-focused program through your college, you are much more likely to get quality educational opportunities than with programs found through random internet searches. Much like choosing a college, be sure these programs work for you and your goals. While they can be fun, they can also be very costly while not offering much in the way of academic advancement or brownie points on your veterinary school application.

Getting Help

Don't underestimate organic chemistry and biochemistry! These are extremely challenging courses. There is no shame in getting a tutor or getting extra help from the professor, and it will make sure you come out of these difficult classes with adequate grades. Nearly everyone struggles with organic chemistry, so don't take it as a sign that you're not meant to be a veterinarian if you need help. Instead, recognize that this is a weak area for you, and take measures to overcome the obstacle. Getting help isn't a sign of weakness, it's a sign of strength, self-awareness, and maturity. Failing to handle this challenge can result in a very poor grade, and that can really hurt your vet school application.

Rounding Out Your Veterinary Experience

As you go through college, you will need to continue to gain veterinary and animal experience. You will also need to have a job. If you can get a job at a small animal or large animal emergency clinic, even if it's just one or two days a week, that will bolster your vet school application significantly. It doesn't matter so much what you do there, whether it's answering the phone or cleaning stalls and kennels. The fact that you spent a lot of time in that environment means that you have a real-world understanding of that side of animal health, and that's important.

Here are a few other places to work that will gain you meaningful experience:

- Small animal vet clinic

- Humane society/SPCA

- Large animal vet clinic or hospital

- University lab working with animals

- Zoo, wildlife habitat, or animal sanctuary

As with all of your experiences, make sure you keep your binder up to date!

Recommendation Letters

One key component to your application packet to vet school is recommendation letters. These carry a lot of weight with the admissions committee! A recommendation letter is a letter written by someone else on your behalf, endorsing you as an applicant and future veterinarian. These are usually written by a veterinarian you've worked for or shadowed, or a professor you've spent a lot of time with. Most applicants have between three and six recommendation letters.

Requesting Letters of Recommendation

Before you get in a hurry to ask someone to write you a recommendation letter for vet school, let's talk about it for a minute. These letters are a big deal, really big. What's said in them counts for a lot, and what's *not* said in them also counts for a lot.

If you ask someone who doesn't really know you to write you a letter, the only thing they have to go on is the interactions you've had with them. For example, we see a lot of letters written by professors who obviously don't know anything about the student. They don't write a great letter for the student, because they don't know what to put in there.

Here's an example of one of these:

> *Dear Admissions Committee,*
>
> *I'm writing to recommend Sally Student for your veterinary program. She attended my organic chemistry class in the fall semester of her sophomore year. She had great attendance, and her grades were good. I'm sure she'll do well in vet school.*

Not a stellar letter. But wait, you say. I just wouldn't include that letter in my packet, that's all. Guess what? In most application systems, you'll never see your recommendation letters. When you start the application process for vet school, you will request recommendation letters through the online application system. The people you ask will receive an email with a link, and that's the end of your part in things. You don't ever get to see the letter they write. Now you see why it's all so important, right? If you made a bad impression, or they don't remember you, they could write you a bad letter, and you wouldn't know.

The same goes for letters from veterinarians. If you work in a vet clinic, and you spend all your time working with Dr. Smith, who is an associate veterinarian, asking Dr. Miller, the practice owner who doesn't really know you, for a letter might not really help you out. You want letters from people who know that you're amazing and motivated and a hard worker, people who are excited to see you succeed. The vets and professors who are your biggest cheerleaders are the ones you want writing your recommendation letters. Here's an example of a not-so-great letter from a veterinarian:

> *My name is Dr. Miller, and I own Mayberry Equine Veterinary Clinic. I'm writing on behalf of Sally Student. Sally shadowed me and both of my associate veterinarians through high school and college, and worked as a tech for one of my associates for a year. I didn't spend much time with her, but from what I can tell, she was a good tech. She has a positive attitude, and everyone seems to like her. I don't know how her work ethic is, as she never worked for me directly. Please call me if you have any questions.*

Also not a stellar letter. Just for contrast, here is a letter from a veterinarian that will get the attention of everyone on the admissions committee:

Dear Admissions Committee,

My name is Dr. Smith, and I am incredibly excited and honored to write this letter of recommendation for Sally Student. I am an associate veterinarian at Mayberry Equine, where I've worked for ten years. In that time, I've seen a lot of people who want to become veterinarians, but I have never had anyone as amazing and energetic as Sally. She is unbelievably intelligent and eager to learn. The energy she brings every day makes her a joy to work with, and her endless questions and relentless commitment to becoming a veterinarian have made me a better veterinarian and teacher. While I hate to lose her as a tech, I have absolutely no doubt that she will be a wonderful veterinarian, and our entire profession will benefit tremendously from having her as a part of it. I am so proud of her, and in awe of her as a human being, and I guarantee that you will be, as well, when you meet her for an interview.

Sally started here as a shadow, and we spent a lot of time together. She was quick to jump in and help, and the emergencies she saw with us didn't scare her away. When she came to work for us, I was excited to have her as my tech. She is very organized, and impressively driven and self-motivated. She has endless enthusiasm, and is a wonderful team member. She has also helped us improve our inventory system, and created tracking processes that make us a better vet clinic.

With my very highest esteem and most sincere intent, I urge you to accept Sally into your vet school program.

See the difference? One letter is essentially just verifying employment or experience, and the other is campaigning on behalf of the applicant. The admissions committee sees a lot of the first kind, and a few of the second kind. If you have two or three fantastic letters like that, the admissions committee will know that you're something special. However, people aren't going to campaign for you unless you give them good reason to. And if Sally moved on to another vet clinic to gain different experiences to help bolster her application, she would need to remind Dr. Smith about what all she did while she was there. That's done with a fact sheet, which we'll talk about momentarily.

Asking people who are not a veterinarian or a professor to write you a letter is okay, but it needs to be a person who knows you and has spent a lot of time with you doing something related to veterinary medicine. For example, if you go to Africa and spend a month working in an animal sanctuary or rehab center, and they are really impressed with you, that might be a good recommendation letter to request. Your hunter/jumper trainer, on the other hand, is *not* someone who should write you a letter unless you spent significant time working for them, not just training with them.

FACT SHEETS

Not everyone has experience writing letters of recommendation, or writing *great* letters. To cover all the bases of a great letter, they'll need some information from you. A great way to make sure they cover all the bases is to make a fact sheet for them. After all, they can't be expected to remember all the pertinent details of what you've done, and when you did it. You'll have to create a custom fact sheet for each person you want a letter from, and here is a list of things that you'll need to include:

- Your name, so they spell it right

- The dates you worked with them

- Some of the key experiences you had there

- Examples of things that demonstrate your eagerness to learn, your work ethic, and your enthusiasm for becoming a veterinarian

There's a certain amount of self-promotion required here, but don't balk at that. You need these people to have all of your best features in the front of their mind when they write the letter, and the only way to make that happen is to list it out for them. Two years might have passed since you spent that time with them, and people forget things. You will have all the information in your vet school binder, of course, but they'll need some help. It's also a good idea to stay in touch with these people as you move on through college, just so they don't forget how amazing you are! This is good practice for building and maintaining relationships, which is a skill you will need for your entire life.

BUILDING RELATIONSHIPS

Aside from the fact sheet, the other thing that will impact the letter they write is the relationship you have with them, and your performance during the time you've spent with them. You have to bring your A game every day when you come to work or class, because the impression you make on that person will have a huge influence on whether or not your application makes it past the first level of screening.

If you have three mediocre recommendation letters from people who aren't convinced that you are the greatest thing ever, you will be at a serious disadvantage to someone else who has three fantastic letters, even if you have better grades and more experience. The opinion of veterinarians as to whether or not you'd be a good veterinarian carries a lot of weight. It's not everything, but it's a lot. So, work very hard to be the best version of you that you can be. Realize that the relationship that you have with your mentors is of supreme importance, and it needs to be legit. Kissing up won't get you there, you have to perform. And finally, don't ask someone for a letter if you're not positive that they will really come through for you. A bad letter is worse than no letter at all.

CHAPTER 7

SOCIAL EXPERIENCE

Social experience is something that you might not think about in terms of being a good veterinarian, but it's a big part of things. When you fill out your vet school application, they're going to ask you about your experiences with volunteering for charitable causes and what sorts of diversity experience that you have. Don't go into this thinking that your amazing animal experience will be enough to carry you past this! Social awareness is a big deal.

Why the fuss?

As a veterinarian, you will be a leader in the community. Not only will people rely on you to help their animals, but you will also be influencing the people who work for you, and the next generation of veterinarians who come to you for experience. As such, it's important that you have a broad understanding of humanity, and not just your particular corner of it.

On the other side of that coin, you will go through college and vet school with a very wide variety of people. Some of them may be very different from you, different culture, different religion, different gender identities, different adversities. Later on, you will have clients and staff/team members who are very different from you, too. Your ability to navigate these differences and build inclusive, meaningful relationships is important.

Gaining Social Awareness

People tend to gravitate to people who are similar to them. It's just the way we're wired. That doesn't mean that we're opposed to people who are different, it just means we're comfortable being around things that we're familiar with.

To gain exposure to people of other cultures, other races and ethnicities, other socio-economic status, you have to make an effort, and do something different. For some, this means volunteering at a homeless shelter or soup kitchen. For others, it might mean working in a Japanese restaurant, or volunteering in a nursing home, reading books or playing cards with elderly people. It can be volunteering at a free animal clinic that provides services for homeless people's animals.

Many young people go on trips abroad, either with a religious organization or a civic or veterinary organization.

These trips can immerse you in a foreign culture for a few weeks, allowing you to see how other people live and interact while you help to improve their lives in some way. These experiences are a great way to broaden your horizons and help others, whether it's by painting houses or vaccinating horses.

In college, you'll likely have access to some cross-cultural clubs or organizations. The purpose of these is to help people meet people of different ethnicities and heritages, and to build relationships and create awareness. Celebrating diversity will make you a better classmate, teammate, veterinarian, and ultimately, a better leader.

Tracking Your Experience

Just like all of your other experiences, you'll need to track your social awareness experiences in your binder. You'll need the same information: names, dates, contact information (if applicable), and what you did.

If you go to Haiti with a group of veterinarians and volunteers to spay and neuter dogs and cats for two weeks, you'll have an experience that falls under several different categories. This would be a diversity experience, a veterinary experience, and a volunteer experience. Which tab do you list it under in your binder? All of them!

When you fill out your vet school application, you'll list

this experience everywhere that it's relevant. Under the veterinary experiences section, focus your description on what you did with the animals. Under the diversity section, talk about your interactions with the Haitian people, and what you learned from them. Don't worry about being redundant, the admissions committee gets it. Remember, they see hundreds of applications every year.

Explaining Your Experience

If you are a middle-class white kid who grew up in a primarily white area, you don't have much diversity experience. That's okay! However, when you are talking about that trip to Haiti on your application, don't try to sell yourself as an expert in diversity. You're not, and the admissions committee knows that. What they're looking for is self-awareness.

It's not important that you know all about people who are different from you. What *is* important is that you realize that you don't know much, and that you're trying to change that. Consider the following two diversity statements:

DIVERSITY STATEMENT A

> *Every summer since I was 13, my family has va-cationed in Jamaica. I have seen lots of Jamaicans*

who work in the hotel, and I also learned that a lot of professional baseball players are from Jamaica. I enjoy listening to their music when we go down to the beach, and my dad always leaves the wait staff a good tip. I've learned that if you are nice and leave them a good tip, they will provide great service to you. They are very nice people if you give them a chance.

Diversity Statement B

I grew up in rural North Carolina, and as a kid, I had very little exposure to people of other cultures or socio-economic backgrounds. I tried to improve my understanding of people with different life experiences by joining the Diversity and Inclusion group in college. I built several lasting friendships during that experience. I also learned that my corner of the world was really small, and there's a lot out there to learn. In addition to D&I, I also volunteered at St. Francis soup kitchen, where I interacted with homeless people and helped them find clothes from the donation shelves. I will continue to seek out opportunities to experience other cultures and build bridges, as I feel I am a more well-rounded person every time I learn something new.

In Statement A, the candidate has been exposed to people from another culture, but they didn't seem to experience any personal growth from the interaction. There is also an element of immaturity and elitism, and both of those things are red flags for the admissions committee.

In Statement B, the candidate's self-awareness is evident, and they expressed a desire to grow in this area. They sought out diversity experiences, rather than observing it through happenstance. This candidate discussed actions taken and lessons learned, which shows maturity and selflessness. While maybe imperfect, Statement B shows a much more suitable candidate.

What if I'm a diverse person?

If you come from an ethnically or culturally diverse background, talk about it! Explain your life experience, what you have learned, and how your diversity will contribute to your career as a veterinarian. Do you speak another language? Does your gender identity cause you to engage with the world in a way that has broadened your understanding of humanity? These are things that the admissions committee wants to know. How have the experiences in your life impacted you, and how will you use that to make the world a more inclusive place?

More Information is Good Information

Your vet school application is an electronic form. It has a series of questions, and you will type in your answers.

This form, which will be made up of your transcripts, your recommendation letters, and your life experiences from your binder, is all that you have to get you past the initial screening so that you can have a face-to-face interview. What you write down is what represents you. Don't hold back! Vet schools aren't looking for robots, they're looking for people. Express yourself. Tell the whole story. Show your personality and character. Don't try to hide who you are, make it a billboard. *This is me! I'm going to be an awesome veterinarian because this is who I am!*

If you try to make yourself inconspicuous and invisible, you will be just that: invisible. You need your electronic document to jump off the screen and grab their attention. You do that by explaining very clearly what you've done to prepare yourself. If you've done twenty things that we've talked about, then you will be clearly more qualified than someone who has done three or four things. Talk about everything you've done, even if it seems inconsequential to you. It might be important to someone on the admissions committee, and that could be the difference of getting an interview, or not getting an interview. You have to advocate for yourself.

Don't rush your way through the essay questions on your vet school application. What you say there is important. Be thoughtful, and have someone else, such as your mentor, read over your work to make sure that you are coming across the way you intend to. Having someone outside your diversity group give you feedback can save you from making unconscious blunders, so seek input from a variety of people. This application is not something you complete in an hour and submit, it's something that you spend years preparing for, and days or weeks perfecting with a team of trusted advisors. Your future depends on it!

CHAPTER 8

ALTERNATE CAREER PATHS: CHANGING YOUR MIND ISN'T QUITTING!

So, you've done a lot of shadowing, and maybe even worked at a veterinary clinic, and you're starting to think that maybe being an equine veterinarian isn't for you, after all. Or maybe you're still at the beginning of your journey, and you aren't sure what you want to do. That's okay! No matter how far you've come down this path, and even if you're in vet school, there are options. You can do a lot of different things with a DVM degree besides work on horses. You can also do a lot of things with horses without a DVM degree.

Many people find through shadowing experiences that they actually like the idea of being a vet tech better than being a veterinarian. That's okay! You can have a very rewarding career as a veterinary assistant, nurse, or technician (they're called different things in different places). You can take classes to become a Certified Veterinary Technician (CVT), and even specialize in a variety of things, such as emergency and critical care, dental care, internal medicine, surgery, anesthesia, physical rehabilitation, and many other areas in both small and large animal. If you decide that this is the career path for you, then all of your experiences leading up to that will be just as relevant, and just as helpful in building your resume.

We're not going to hit this in-depth, but here is a short list of career fields that are related to horses or the DVM degree in some way. It's not an all-inclusive list by any means. We're just trying to show you that going down the pre-vet track doesn't limit your options to just one or two things. Even if you decide not to go to vet school at all, there are a wide variety of things you can do with horses in the academic world, the feed and health industry, and other places.

Veterinary Careers

- Veterinarian for USDA, APHIS, or other government agencies

- Technical Services veterinarian for pharmaceutical, feed, or animal health industries

- Teaching from community colleges to graduate schools

- Research in just about any science field, and even some education and business fields

- Corporate veterinarian (project managers and policy directors for pharmaceutical companies)

Non-Veterinary Careers

- Animal Science Professor (this can cover a wide range of specialties)

- Geneticist (this is an emerging and rapidly growing area)

- Nutritionist (feed companies like Purina and Nutrena employ lots of equine nutritionists)

- County Extension Agent/Specialist

- Certified Veterinary Technician

- Behaviorist (research scientists who study horse behavior)

- Sales Rep for feed, pharmaceutical, or animal health businesses

- Biomechanist (research scientists who study how horses move)

- Researcher in one of the many, many areas of scientific study

When you get to college, you'll find a whole world of research science you never knew existed. You can participate as a student in many of these projects, and that will open other doors for you into the world of research science. There is a lot of research taking place regarding nearly every aspect of equine health and behavior.

Genetic testing in horses is an exploding market. There are several companies who do this, as well as universities, and the field is still in the early stages of development. If you decide genetics is your thing, there is a way to tie it into horses!

There are many, many things you can do in the world of equine science. Every feed company employs countless veterinarians and non-veterinarians. Pharmaceutical companies, who make the drugs we use on horses, have tons of jobs for both veterinarians and non-veterinarians. If you love veterinary medicine, but you can't be a general practitioner for some reason, you can still find a challenging, fulfilling career in a related field.

Changing your mind isn't quitting, it's making an intelligent decision based on new information. Do what's right for you.

CHAPTER 9

WORKING FOR EXPERIENCE

Many college graduates don't get accepted into vet school on their first try. Some don't make it on their second try. Or third. That's okay! In many ways, having a year or two between college and vet school can be a huge advantage to you in the long run. It's what you do with that time that matters.

If you want to become an equine veterinarian, then the best thing you can do with a free year is to work as a technician or veterinary assistant at an equine clinic or hospital. Depending on where you live, you might have to move for a year to make this happen, but the experience you gain will be worth it. Not only will you learn things that will help you get through vet school, but the experience itself might be what gets you into vet school on your next try.

If you've done the groundwork through high school and college, then you know all of the equine veterinarians in your area that you might get a job with. You've probably shadowed most of them and worked part-time for some of them. Because you've already done that, you know which ones will give you the best experience, and you already have a foot in the door. Hopefully you made a great impression on them the last time you were there, and they're eager to have you back. Yes, that really happens!

If we were to create a perfect scenario for you, it would be that you get to work in two places: a big referral hospital with lots of doctors, lots of staff, and lots of horses, and a small practice with two or three doctors. Our goal would be that you become intimately familiar with life inside both practices, as they are very different places. At the end of a year, you will know for sure if you still want to be an equine veterinarian. If the answer is no, after living it for a year, day in and day out, then that was the best year you'll ever spend learning something. Many people find out that they were meant for other things, and that's incredibly important to know about yourself. As we've said before, you want to find this out *before* you go to vet school, not after.

Hands-On Experience

If you've shadowed a lot of veterinarians through high school and college, and taken good notes in your vet school binder, then you know the places where you'll get the best experience in your area. See how it's all coming together? The more places you shadowed, the better your list is, and the easier your job hunt will be.

Some equine practices are well-known for being great places to work, and getting a job there can be challenging. Being an awesome shadow is the number one way to get your foot in the door for a job. When you are shadowing a vet, you're sizing them up as a potential future employer. At the same time, they're sizing you up as a potential future employee. If you are eager to learn, highly self-motivated about jumping in and doing what needs to be done, and you really fit in with the team, they've noticed! And if you spent a lot of time sitting around scrolling through social media back when you were a shadow, they noticed that, too. So, treat every shadow experience as a working job interview.

When you're interviewing for a job, be open and upfront about what your goals are. You may be afraid that they won't want to hire you if you're only planning to be there for a year, but that's not always true. Many veterinarians make it a point to support young people on a vet school track. It will also impact the kind of experience you have there. If they don't know you're trying to go to vet school, then they probably won't go out of their way to teach you things outside of your tech duties.

If you're working for an ambulatory veterinarian, you'll be spending a lot of time riding around in the vet truck. This is a golden opportunity that many people would kill for (not literally). You will have one-on-one time with a veterinarian every day, sometimes several hours of it. While the vet will be doing a variety of things, such as typing medical notes, calling and texting clients, and so on, there will still be lots of time to talk. Don't waste this time!

The vet you work for will be your best resource for knowledge and experience, and you want to get as much of both as you possibly can. You will also need this vet to write you a letter of recommendation for vet school, and you need to convince them that you are the greatest candidate for vet school that has come along since they were there themselves. How do you do that? By being a great tech, and a great student. Ask lots of questions. Do every single thing they'll let you do. Ask them to teach you how to tube a horse, how to insert a catheter, what they see on the ultrasound, why they give vaccines where they do, and a million other things. Demonstrate what you've learned every chance you get. If you get two hours a day with that vet for a year, make it your goal to learn everything possible from them in that year, and make sure they know that's your goal.

If the practice has more than one veterinarian, then you should do everything we just talked about with all of them that you have access to. If you can get two or three very strong recommendation letters from doctors in the same practice, that will really help you on your vet school application. In addition to experience, getting those letters is one of your top priorities. Recommendation letters from veterinarians carry more weight than letters from non-veterinarians, simply because vets know what it really takes to be a vet, and they can often tell better than other people if you have it.

CHAPTER 10

APPLYING TO VET SCHOOL

Different vet schools have different applications, but they are all generally interested in the same things. What have you done to prepare yourself? Do you know what you're getting into? Do you have what it takes to be a good veterinarian? We've talked all about gaining animal, work, and veterinary experience. Now we're going to talk about how to present yourself and your experiences.

The Application

There is a general veterinary school application that is the same for every school in the United States and Canada, and for a long list of international schools as well. This application is done through the Veterinary Medical College Application Service (VMCAS). Many of the vet schools will also have supplementary application materials and fees along with the general application. Many of these supplemental materials can be done along with your main VMCAS, but some schools require a separate supplemental application.

Long before you begin the application itself, research the schools. It costs money to apply to vet school, and VMCAS charges by the number of schools you apply to. Applying to all of them isn't the best financial plan. You always have the best chance of admission, and the best tuition rate, at your in-state school, so make sure that one is on your list. For out-of-state schools there are several important factors to research: number of seats available for out-of-state students, number of those seats not pledged to a particular state, tuition for out-of-state students, cost of living, and whether or not you can change status to in-state during the program.

As an example, let's look at the difference being an in-state vs. an out-of-state student makes for your application to the University of Florida. The in-state tuition for Florida would be about $29,000 per year as of the release date of this book (2020), vs. $45,000 for out-of-state. There are 94 seats for in-state students out of an applicant pool of 390 people. There are 26 slots for out-of-state with an applicant pool of a whopping 884 people. That's a big difference in your chances of getting in and your tuition. These are important considerations! While this may be time consuming, this information is readily available on the VMCAS website. Take the time to evaluate each college you are considering applying to, and talk with veterinarians you know to get additional insider information.

The application itself consists of three major parts: information about you, your transcripts, and essay questions. The section with information about you is going to be so much simpler because of the binder you've used to keep track of all your veterinary experience. This is where you will put in all your jobs, research, volunteer, and veterinary experiences. You will also fill out all your college coursework in the transcript section. One caveat is to make sure your transcripts arrive at VMCAS. Don't take it for granted that you've requested them, and so they've been sent.

Now onto the essay questions. The most important thing to consider when reading these questions is *why*. Why are these particular questions being asked? Put yourself in the position of the admissions committee members. This is their chance to get to know you. They want to know they are letting someone into their program who will be teachable, employable, and a good representative for the school. Approach the questions with this in mind. Once you have written your essays, have someone evaluate them for you. Ask for very critical feedback. You only have a few paragraphs to make this impression. Rewrite your essay with the feedback you've gotten, and then proofread it. If English isn't your first language, and you worry about your writing skills, that's okay! These essays aren't harshly judged on perfect grammar. However, obvious typos can be taken as a sign that you aren't paying attention to important details. Remember, you're applying for veterinary school. Not noticing that you typed *hte* instead of *the*, indicates you may not notice important things about patients in the future.

For supplemental applications, follow the same essay guidelines. There are reasons these particular questions are being asked. Put yourself in the place of an admissions committee member.

The Interview

Each school has a slightly different interview style, but in general they want to know that you can speak to other people in a high stress environment. Being nervous is absolutely okay. Being unable to communicate because of those nerves is not. Most of the schools will interview you with a few members of the admissions committee. This means you will need to be comfortable being the interviewee with more than one interviewer. The best way to do this is practice, practice, practice. Get your friends together for practice interviews. In many ways, it can be much more difficult to interview with people you know than people you don't which is good prep for your vet school interview.

In general, interviewers will be asking you about your work and school history, with some schools adding behavioral interview questions. Did you get a less than ideal grade in Organic Chemistry? Be prepared to discuss why that happened, and what you learned about yourself in the process. Look through your binder to make sure you remember all the places you've worked and volunteered. Go back to any research you were involved in. Think about what you learned at each one, and how that impacts your future as a veterinarian. This will allow you to go in depth on a simple question like, "Tell me about your time at XYZ Equine Clinic." This shows maturity, and a willingness to look beyond the simple answer. Both are important things in veterinary school, and beyond.

Behavioral questions are trickier. These are questions like, *Tell me about your biggest failure, and how you handled it.* They require you to be very self-aware. There are many behavioral interview resources available. One we like is *Ideal Team Player* by Patrick Lencioni. This is a book and website. Both discuss what's really important to employers, and the same concepts can be applied to veterinarians. Those friends who helped you go over your history can help you with this section, too.

At some point in your application or interview process it is very likely you'll get asked why you want to be a veterinarian. Now is the time to think about your answer.

Because I like animals, is never a good enough answer, and yet it's the single most common answer. Consider your motivations for pursuing veterinary medicine, and equine medicine in particular. Having a solid answer for this question will put you ahead of many other applicants.

There are some excellent resources available to help you prepare for your interview. One of these is StudentDoctorNetwork.net. People report their interview experiences here, which allows you a peek at how different schools that you are considering handle the interview process. Seek out interviewing insights from the vets you've shadowed, and work on your communication and public speaking skills. And again, practice, practice, practice getting interviewed!

CHAPTER 11

STUDENT LOANS

Student debt is a topic of many discussions these days. Tuition is higher than ever before, as is the cost of living. Many students graduate from vet school with $200,000, $300,000, and even $400,000 in debt. To be clear, this is just the cost of vet school. Your undergrad debt is a separate thing. Let's take a look at how that happens.

Vet school tuition is expensive, and it's not likely to get cheaper. However, there are a lot of other things that contribute to your student debt. Housing, food, transportation, and spending money can all end up being borrowed. When you've been in college for five or six years with this student debt elephant following you around, it's easy to get numb to it, and stop taking it seriously. *It's such a huge number already, so what does it matter if I add another $10,000 to it? I might as well be able to live decently while I'm here.* You do that once. At first, it makes you queasy, but after a year goes by, it doesn't even faze you anymore. You do it again. And maybe again.

We're going to do some math here. We're using a student loan calculator, available free online. If you add $10,000 to your loan, it will accumulate $5,839 in interest over twenty years at 5% interest. If your interest rate is 6%, that becomes $7,194. That's just the interest, and just on the extra $10,000 you borrowed. That means if you're paying $10 for something using student loan money, you're really paying $15- $17. If you spend $100, you're really spending $150 - $170. Don't forget that.

If you're able to work through college and earn some money, you can reverse that scenario. Paying for your food, gas, coffee, and clothes out of your paycheck will save you thousands of dollars. Cutting the amount you borrow by $40,000 will save you $60K - $70K over the life of the loan. That's a really big deal! But we're getting ahead of ourselves. We'll talk about that more in a bit.

Understanding the System

There are several different ways that student loan repayment plans can work. These change from time to time, so don't make your financial plans based on what we have here. Do your homework and see what the current options are. Once you graduate vet school, you will decide which plan is best for you and lock it in.

There are plans that allow you to pay back your student loan over either 10 or 20 years. Both of these plans have pros and cons.

10 Year Plan:

Pros: Pay less interest. Loan paid off after 10 years.

Cons: High monthly payment.

20 Year Plan:

Pros: Lower monthly payment.

Cons: Pay more interest. Making payments for 20 years.

Either of these plans can be a good choice if your total debt is relatively small.

Debt Forgiveness/ Pay As You Earn (PAYE) Plans

In contrast to the complete payment plans, we have the student debt forgiveness plans, such as PAYE. The way these work is that instead of paying back your entire loan, you make monthly payments based on how much money you earn each year. These payments last for 20 years. At the end of the 20 years, whatever amount of your debt that hasn't been paid off gets forgiven. Sounds great, right? There's a catch: You have to pay income tax on the amount that's forgiven. Income tax is around 25% or a bit more. Your loan is accumulating interest all this time, too.

How do you know which plan makes the most sense? You have to do some math. We'll do some together in this example so you can see.

10 Year and 20 Year Full Repayment Plans

The best way to pay the least amount of interest, and therefore, the least amount of money overall for your student loans, is to take the 10 Year Plan. The amount of interest money you'll save is staggering. Unfortunately, so is the monthly payment. As you'll see in our budget section below, making a $2,000 payment each month is very difficult to maintain. However, there are a lot of variables, and if you wind up with a job that allows you enough income to make these payments, you'll save anywhere from $50K to $100K, and that's enough for a nice car, or a down payment on a house. The following table shows monthly payments, interest, and total payouts for various loan amounts.

These were calculated at 5% interest. If your interest rate is higher, you'll pay more. If it's lower, you'll pay less.

	10 Year Loan, Normal Payback		
Total Loan Amount	Interest at 5%	Monthly Payment (10 years)	Total Payment
$ 150,000.00	$ 40,918.00	$ 1,591.00	$ 190,918.00
$ 200,000.00	$ 54,557.00	$ 2,121.00	$ 254,557.00
$ 250,000.00	$ 68,197.00	$ 2,651.00	$ 318,197.00
$ 300,000.00	$ 81,836.00	$ 3,181.00	$ 381,836.00
$ 350,000.00	$ 95,475.00	$ 3,712.00	$ 445,475.00

The other option that is currently available is the 20 Year Plan. These options change with time, so do your homework to find out what your specific options are. For the purposes of familiarizing you with student loans, the 10 and 20 Year Plans work great, as you'll be able to see the difference that time and interest make.

With a twenty-year loan, your monthly payment is lower. The tradeoff is that you will pay more interest, because it's spread over twice as many years. In the table below, you'll see the same options as the ten-year loan table, calculated at 5% interest.

	20 Year Loan, Normal Payback		
Total Loan Amount	Interest at 5%	Monthly Payment (20 years)	Total Payment
$ 150,000.00	$ 87,584.00	$ 990.00	$ 237,584.00
$ 200,000.00	$ 116,779.00	$ 1,320.00	$ 316,779.00
$ 250,000.00	$ 145,973.00	$ 1,649.00	$ 395,973.00
$ 300,000.00	$ 175,168.00	$ 1,979.00	$ 475,168.00
$ 350,000.00	$ 204,363.00	$ 2,309.00	$ 554,363.00

Pay As You Earn (PAYE) Plans

As you'll see in the tables below, the monthly payments for PAYE loans are much smaller than the full repayment loans. That can be misleading, so don't jump to conclusions! Along with the smaller monthly payment, you also have a big tax payment that has to be made at the twenty-year mark. That's a factor on your monthly budget, because you'll need to save anywhere from $100 to $400 every month for twenty years to able to pay the tax bill at the end.

The amount of your monthly payment is calculated each year based on your tax returns from the year before. That means your payment amount can go up and down, along with the amount of tax you'll owe at the end. The following table shows the tax payments for various loan amounts based on a 5% interest rate, and it assumes that you are making $75K per year, and you file your taxes as a single person.

Monthly payment, based on $75K Salary and single income household $700					Total Payout over 20 Years $ 168,000.00	
PAYE, Based on Single Income Household and $75K Income (Payment is 15% of Discretionary Income)						
Loan Amount	Interest Accrued at 5%	Amount Paid	Amount forgiven	Tax owed (balloon payment)	Total Payout with Tax	
$ 150,000.00	$ 87,584.00	$ 168,000.00	$ 69,584.00	$ 17,396.00	$ 185,396.00	
$ 200,000.00	$ 136,779.00	$ 168,000.00	$ 148,779.00	$ 37,194.75	$ 205,194.75	
$ 250,000.00	$ 145,973.00	$ 168,000.00	$ 227,973.00	$ 56,993.25	$ 224,993.25	
$ 300,000.00	$ 175,168.00	$ 168,000.00	$ 307,168.00	$ 76,792.00	$ 244,792.00	
$ 350,000.00	$ 204,363.00	$ 168,000.00	$ 386,363.00	$ 96,590.75	$ 264,590.75	

With those conditions, your payment would be about $700 a month. If your loan is $200,000, you'll also need to save an additional $150 a month for your tax bill.

As you make more money, your monthly payment will go up. That's not all bad! As you pay more on your loan, your final tax payment gets smaller. The table below shows those same loans but based on your annual income at $100K instead of $75K. Your monthly payment is now $1,025 but look at your tax amount.

Monthly payment, based on $100,000 Salary and single income household					Total Payout over 20 Years	
	$1,025				$ 246,000.00	
	PAYE, Based on Single Income Household and $100,000 Income (Payment is 15% of Discretionary Income)					
Loan Amount	Interest Accrued at 5%	Amount Paid	Amount forgiven	Tax owed (balloon payment)	Total Payout with Tax	
$ 150,000.00	$ 87,584.00	$ 246,000.00	$	$ -	$ 237,584.00	
$ 200,000.00	$ 116,779.00	$ 246,000.00	$ 70,779.00	$ 17,694.75	$ 263,694.75	
$ 250,000.00	$ 149,973.00	$ 246,000.00	$ 149,973.00	$ 37,493.25	$ 283,493.25	
$ 300,000.00	$ 175,168.00	$ 246,000.00	$ 229,168.00	$ 57,292.00	$ 303,292.00	
$ 350,000.00	$ 204,363.00	$ 246,000.00	$ 308,363.00	$ 77,090.75	$ 323,090.75	

As you can see, the amount forgiven and tax owed for the $150,000 line are blank. That's because you'll pay off the loan before you get to the 20-year mark if you pay $1,025 every month. If you look back at the table for the 20 Year Full Repayment plan, you'll see that the monthly payment for $150,000 is $990. In this particular case, it makes more sense to do the full repayment plan.

Keep in mind that these tables are calculating rates with the assumption that you will make the exact same amount of money every year for twenty years, and that you will always be in a single-income household. They also assume the interest rate for your loan will be 5%, and that might not be true. Your specific payment will vary from year to year, and the amount of tax you have to pay at the end is difficult to project because of that. It's best to err on the side of caution and save more than you think you'll need.

Another thing to consider with PAYE plans is unusual circumstances. If you inherit money, or sell your practice, or write a best-selling book, those things all count as income. You might sell your practice fifteen years down the road for a million dollars. Guess what? Your loan payments the following year are going to go through the roof as a result of that. And selling your practice for a million doesn't mean that you'll have a million to play with. You'll likely have business loans to pay off with it. You might have enough left over to pay off your student loan, but then again, you might not. These situations happen all the time in the real world. That doesn't mean you shouldn't choose a PAYE plan, but it does mean you need to carefully consider how your financial decisions will impact your loan payments.

Monthly Budget with Student Loans

Let's look forward in time and try to put this in terms that make sense. You're out of vet school (congratulations, Doctor!). You have a job and a life, and things are good. Let's look at your monthly budget.

	Sample Budget				$75K	$100K
Monthly Bills	$			Monthly Income		
Rent	$ 1,000.00			Paycheck	$ 6,250.00	$ 8,333.00
Car payment	$ 500.00			less tax at 25%	$ 1,562.00	$ 2,083.00
Stdnt Ln Undergrad		(insert your payment here)				
Stdnt Ln Vet Sch		(insert your payment here)				
Car insurance	$ 200.00			Total Income	$ 4,688.00	$ 6,250.00
Food	$ 800.00					
Gas	$ 100.00					
Electricity	$ 200.00					
Phone	$ 100.00					
Internet	$ 100.00					
Health insurance	$ 500.00					
Savings for taxes		(if on PAYE plan)				
Misc	$ 200.00					
Total Expenses	$ 3,700.00	(plus loan payment and tax savings)				

We're making some assumptions here, of course. First, this assumes you're single, and living alone. Next, if you're a horse person, it's likely that you have a horse. Or more than one. We didn't include any of the costs associated with that. We also assume you're living fairly frugally, with no cable tv, and very few extravagances. And a very important omission on this budget is a contribution to a retirement plan. You'll definitely need one of those! For the purposes of keeping our sample budget simple, we went minimal.

The average pay for an equine veterinarian in the US is around $75,000 a year. After taxes and withholdings, that leaves you about $4,500 a month. Average means that some make more than that, but some also make less. Keep in mind that everyone goes into the workforce expecting to be on the upper half of that pay range, but only half actually end up there. In many places where the wages are low, the cost of living is also lower, so don't panic! Your rent might only be $600 a month. On the flip side of that, higher income areas usually cost more to live in. Having a higher wage doesn't always mean more money at the end of the month!

You might not have to make a car payment right away, but at some point, you're going to have to buy a new(er) car. Depending on where you work, health insurance might be provided for you, so that could save you $500 a month. If you have a roommate or a spouse, you can split some of the bills, so that will help.

Now let's look back at the monthly payment tables above and try to figure out what makes sense on our budget, and what doesn't. There are a lot of variables here, and every person's situation is going to be different, so keep that in mind. For this example, let's say you did a great job with scholarships and jobs, and you don't have any debt from undergrad. Then you worked for a year to get experience, and you were smart about your spending in vet school. Your total debt is $200,000.

If we look back up at our tables, we can see that it's significantly cheaper to take the PAYE option, regardless of how much money you make. If your debt was $150,000, it would be the other way around.

The less you borrow in college and vet school, the smaller those student loan numbers will be. Keep in mind that your interest rate could be higher, too, and a 1% increase in interest over 20 years will make a big impact on your loan. Look at how much the interest changes in the table below.

Loan Amount	5% Interest	6% Interest	7% Interest
$ 200,000.00	$ 116,779.00	$ 143,887.00	$ 172,143.00
$ 300,000.00	$ 175,168.00	$ 215,830.00	$ 258,215.00

Borrowing Less, Paying Less

While the excitement of going off to college and being out on your own is a wonderful feeling, it's important to enjoy it responsibly, rather than digging a hole that you'll spend the next twenty years trying to climb out of. Living at home with your parents in college, or with roommates that may not be the easiest to live with, can be tough, but if you keep your focus on your goals, it will allow you a lot more breathing room once you're out in the working world. You can also impact these things with the money you earn working in high school and college. Having a job in vet school is almost impossible, but you can minimize your student loans and maximize your work experience leading up to that point and showing your ability to do that counts for a lot on your vet school application.

The number one thing you can do to reduce your student loans is go to a cheaper school for your undergrad degree. If you can take college classes in high school and graduate with an associate's degree, then you only need two years of school to get your bachelor's degree. Rather than going to the big state school to do that, look at some of the smaller colleges in your area. If you can keep living at home with your parents while you work on your undergrad degree at a small school, you might even be able to pay for it with the money you earn working through college. That would put you at a debt level of zero going into vet school, which is the ideal situation.

Don't try to figure it out on your own

One of the great things about going through this process is that there are a lot of resources for you to use. You don't have to try to figure it all out on your own. You can talk to the veterinarians you shadow, and find out what their experience has been. The younger they are, the more relevant their student loan experience will be to you. Talking things over with your family can be helpful, especially if they know a financial or accounting professional who can advise you. Your college will have a variety of resources as well. The more information you gather, the better prepared you'll be to make the decision that's right for you.

CHAPTER 12

EXTERNSHIPS AND INTERNSHIPS

Externships

While you're in vet school, you'll have the opportunity to be an extern. This is a rotation in a veterinary clinic or hospital that typically lasts 2-4 weeks. It's important to go on as many of these as you can. Not only will it bolster your education as a veterinarian, it will also help you find more potential places to get an internship. This is also the beginning of your resume for real-world jobs.

Just like you've been doing since high school, externships are a chance to gain experience, and shop for future employers. As an extern, you'll get to do more things than you could as a shadow. This is a chance to get hands-on and get comfortable doing various things to horses. Believe it or not, you won't get a lot of hands-on experiences in most vet schools. So, it's important to take every opportunity you get to stick a needle in a horse, or palpate one, or perform a dental float.

As we mentioned earlier in the book, you're considering each place you go as a potential place to intern or work as a vet in the future, and they're considering you for an internship or a job later. The impression you make in that externship period is important. By now, you should be a pro at being a pro, but it's worth mentioning again. If you're a bad extern, you won't get a chance to be an intern there.

Some vet students do twenty or thirty externships over the course of their four years. Some only do two or three. When you start applying for internships, your experience with externships is part of the selection process, and equine hospitals don't have time to employ interns who have little or no experience. So, don't take externships lightly!

Internships

Internships are not a requirement to become an equine veterinarian. That being said, the absolute best thing you can do for yourself once you graduate vet school is do an internship. That one year of working in a big equine hospital somewhere, even if that's not at all what you want to do long-term, will set you up for success for the rest of your career. It will also help launch your career.

When you graduate vet school, you'll have a head crammed full of knowledge, and absolutely no idea of how to go be an equine veterinarian. As an intern in a busy hospital, you'll have a mentor (probably several) that will show you the ropes, and you'll get five years' worth of experience in one year, due to the workload. The confidence that comes with that experience is what will make you a great veterinarian and allow you to hit the ground running.

Most equine veterinarians don't want to hire someone fresh out of vet school with no experience. They were there once, themselves, and they know how much you need to learn before you'll be able to start being a productive team member. An internship will make you a desirable, experienced veterinarian, and that will open many more doors for you.

In vet school, you'll be surrounded by students who are going to be small animal veterinarians. Many of them won't do an internship, and they'll make you question the validity of doing one, yourself. They'll talk about how much money they're going to earn their first year out, and you'll know that interns don't make near that much, and that might mess with your head. Don't listen to them!

There are several differences between their future and yours. For one, they're going to work in a clinic that probably has three or four doctors, and they'll see thirty patients a day, with a mentor guiding them. In equine medicine, it doesn't work that way at all. An equine general practice can't afford to spend a year teaching you. They only see five or six horses a day, as opposed to the thirty dogs and cats the small animal vets are seeing. That's far less income for the practice, and far less training for a new veterinarian.

If you do some quick math, you'll realize that your small animal classmates will be getting five times as much experience as you are every day, simply based on caseload. So, they can get by without an internship, although it's still in their best interests to do one. For you, as an equine veterinarian, it's almost not an option to skip this step. Many young vets do, and most of them regret it. So do the practices that hire them.

One of the great things about doing an internship is your exposure to emergency medicine. Your ability to work up a colic at the end of your internship will be stellar, and as an equine general practitioner, you'll need those skills on a regular basis to know if you're going to treat a horse or refer it to a hospital. This skill is critical, because lives hang in the balance. If you skip the internship part and go straight to work, and you've only seen six colics in the last six months instead of the two or three hundred that you'd have seen during an internship, you probably won't know how serious something is or isn't. It doesn't take very many mistakes for you to get a bad reputation among horse owners in your area, and once that happens, you might as well move somewhere else.

Building Your Resume

When it's time to apply for your first job as a full-fledged veterinarian, there are only a few things that will be on your resume: where you went to school, how many externships you did, and where you interned. Remember, all the other vets who graduated the same year you did from all the vet schools across the country are now competing with you for whatever jobs are available.

If you've used all the tools in this book, you have a tremendous advantage over most of your classmates. You are organized, experienced, and confident. You have great communication skills. You're self-aware and have been working on your weak areas since high school. And even though you're just coming off your internship, you've got years of veterinary experience, and you know how to be a great part of a great team. You've got customer service skills, you're self-motivated, and you're not afraid to jump in and try something new. Make sure you talk about these things! This is what sets you apart from the crowd, so use it.

COVER LETTERS

When you apply for internships, and later, for jobs, you'll likely have to write a cover letter to go with your resume. The cover letter is your opportunity to jump up and down, waving a flag and honking your horn. This is your tool for getting noticed: don't waste it! As a veterinary practice owner, we've seen hundreds of resumes and cover letters. The ones who don't display any personality don't get much attention.

Here's a rule of thumb to remember: People who want to blend into the crowd and remain unnoticed are generally successful in doing so. People who want to stick out of the crowd are also usually successful in doing so. If you are trying to get a job, and you're competing with others who have the same resume as you, then you need to stick out of the crowd!

Don't misrepresent yourself, but don't be afraid to show your personality in your cover letter. As practice owners, we're not hiring robots, we're hiring people. We want to hire a doctor that our clients are going to like and accept and build a relationship with. We're hiring a doctor who needs to fit into our team without personality conflicts.

Here's an example of a bad cover letter:

Dear hiring manager,

My name is Dr. Wilson, and I'm a 2018 graduate of the UF Vet School. As you'll see in my resume, I did an internship at Jackson Equine Emergency Center. I'm experienced in colic management and injury management, and I will be an asset to your veterinary clinic. Thank you for your time and consideration.

Here's an example of a good cover letter:

Dear Dr. Smith and the Oakvale Equine Team,

I am very excited to be applying for the associate veterinarian position at Oakvale! I have read your entire website and all your Facebook and Google reviews, and I can tell that Oakvale is a fun place to work and you have a great client base who loves you! That's really important to me.

I've only been a veterinarian for a year, but I've got over two thousand hours of experience in veterinary clinics (not counting my one-year internship), and I have seen what the quality of life is like for good and bad teams. I'm a very positive and engaging person, and I thrive in an environment that values great relationships, both within the team and with the clients.

I've done my homework on you and your clinic, and I know that you are a mentor who is highly valued by everyone you've worked with over the years. I'm seeking that mentorship, as I have a lot to learn, and I want to become the best version of me that I can. I had a wonderful experience in my internship at Jackson Equine Emergency Center, and I want a position that will allow me to continue to learn and grow, both as a doctor and as a person.

I'm a lifelong equestrian, and my 15 years of experience in dressage and showing hunters has given me the ability to connect with horse people on a high level. I understand crazy horse people, because I am one! My OTTB is the love of my life, and I'm looking forward to finding a new training barn to get established with. I believe that I can be a great ambassador for the vet clinic in this way.

Please don't consider the coffee and brownies that I bring to my interview as a form of bribery! I prefer to consider them a token of my appreciation for your time and consideration of me as a potential team member. Please call me at your convenience with any questions!

A good cover letter should reflect your personality, show that you've researched the clinic you're applying to, and it should be custom-crafted, rather than being a form letter. Let them know you did your homework, and what draws you to their clinic. If you're energetic and fun, let that show in your writing! And while most of this process is about showcasing your strengths, volunteering a weak area that you are actively working on says a lot about your self-awareness and your confidence. It takes confidence to talk about your weaknesses, and while everyone has weaknesses, trying to hide them shows your insecurities, not your strength. This letter doesn't highlight a particular weak area, but discusses the desire to learn and grow, and the need for a great mentor.

This should go without saying, but we'll say it anyway: BE HONEST! Job hunting is a lot like dating: the last thing you want to find out six months from now is that all the stuff they told you was a lie. This goes both ways; the vet clinic wants to know the real you, and you want to know the real them. If you are honest and open, and it turns out that you don't fit in, then it isn't the right place for you. That's okay! It doesn't mean there's anything wrong with you or them. Sometimes people just aren't a good match for each other. Again, it's a lot like dating. You can't force it to work out.

CHAPTER 13

CONCLUSION

If you've read this whole book, then you have a pretty good idea of what you need to do. You're probably a little overwhelmed, too! That's a normal response to a seemingly impossible task. Remember, you eat a huge casserole the same way you eat a carrot: one bite at a time. You walk a thousand miles the same way you walk across the room: one step at a time. You don't have to do all this stuff at once. It's a lot, there's no denying that, but others have done it, and you can, too.

You'll probably want to refer back to this book more than once. You can't remember everything on your first time through, and it's not meant to be used that way. Use it as a manual and refer to it often.

It's important to remember that this is your journey. It's not going to be perfect, it's not going to be exactly like someone else's journey, and that's okay. You have a map, and you know the waypoints you need to hit along the way to your destination. How you get from one waypoint to the next is up to you. The key is to avoid getting stuck when you come to an obstacle. There will always be obstacles in life. You have to learn how to use your resources and determination to overcome each one as they come. Every obstacle you encounter is an opportunity to learn and grow, and as you overcome them, you will gain confidence and wisdom.

Be the driver on your journey, not a passenger!

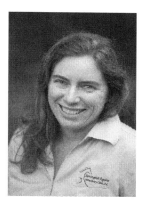

Dr. Erica Lacher is a 2001 graduate of the University of Florida's College of Veterinary Medicine, and the owner of Springhill Equine Veterinary Clinic in Newberry, Florida. In addition to practicing medicine, she is also an author, blogger, and podcaster. Her podcast, *Straight from the Horse Doctor's Mouth,* is popular among horse owners worldwide. She enjoys competing in show jumping with her horses, and spending time outdoors with her husband.

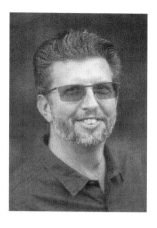

Justin B. Long is a self-embracing nerd who loves crunching numbers, researching interesting things, and listening to podcasts, in addition to reading loads of books. By day he is the CFO of Springhill Equine Veterinary Clinic, and by night he is an author and podcaster. He lives near Gainesville, Florida on a small farm with his incredible wife, 7 horses, 5 cats, 2 donkeys, 2 dogs, and a sheep named Gerald.

Printed in Great Britain
by Amazon

67773408R00083